!

REGROWING HAIR
NATURALLY

REGROWING HAIR
NATURALLY

EFFECTIVE REMEDIES and NATURAL TREATMENTS
for MEN and WOMEN
with ALOPECIA AREATA, ALOPECIA ANDROGENETICA,
TELOGEN EFFLUVIUM and OTHER HAIR LOSS PROBLEMS

Revised Edition

VERA PEIFFER

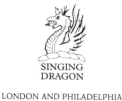

SINGING
DRAGON

LONDON AND PHILADELPHIA

This edition published in 2013
by Singing Dragon
an imprint of Jessica Kingsley Publishers
116 Pentonville Road
London N1 9JB, UK
and
400 Market Street, Suite 400
Philadelphia, PA 19106, USA

www.singingdragon.com

Library of Congress Cataloging in Publication Data
Peiffer, Vera.
  Regrowing hair naturally : effective remedies and natural treatments for men and women with alopecia areata, alopecia androgenetica, telogen effluvium and other hair loss problems / Vera Peiffer.
    pages cm
  Includes index.
  ISBN 978-1-84819-139-6 (alk. paper)
  1. Baldness--Popular works. 2. Baldness--Alternative treatment--Popular works. 3. Hair--Care and hygiene--Popular works. I. Title.
  RL155.P45 2013
  616.5'46--dc23
                                2012051113

British Library Cataloguing in Publication Data
A CIP catalogue record for this book is available from the British Library

ISBN 978 1 84819 139 6
eISBN 978 0 85701 118 3

Printed and bound in Great Britain

CONTENTS

INTRODUCTION OR WHO IS THAT WOMAN ANYWAY?

Imagine waking up one morning and finding a lot of hair on your pillow. As you look at your reflection in the mirror, you notice that your hair looks considerably thinner. Or you are washing your hair one day and notice a small bald patch on your head. You think you have knocked yourself and it will go away, but it doesn't. It gets bigger. Every time you wash your hair, you see masses of hairs drifting off down the plughole. You hardly dare touch your hair because whatever you touch comes off in your hand. Or even worse, imagine going to bed one evening with a full head of hair and waking up the next morning to find that all your hair has fallen out in the night.

If you bought this book for yourself, you will be only too familiar with one of the above situations. Losing some or all of your hair is an intensely traumatic experience.

When I was 14, I discovered a small bald patch on my head which slowly became bigger. My mother took me to see various doctors and dermatologists, but none of them seemed to know why it was happening or what could be done. They gave me some UVA treatment, but that didn't help. Finally, I saw a professor of dermatology who prescribed steroid tablets. I put on a lot of weight, but hairwise, nothing happened. After a year or so, I went on to have steroid injections into the scalp. These were quite painful, and I was also very afraid of needles at the time. I got very stressed, and as a result, my hair suddenly began to fall out really fast. I quickly developed more bald patches all over my head which I could no longer cover with my remaining hair.

I was devastated when I realised that I had to start wearing a wig to cover my baldness. I could not believe what was happening to me, and nothing seemed to stop the hair from falling out. Within another few months, I had lost all the hair on my head. Within another six months, the hair on my entire body had fallen out. At school, other kids started to shun me or make hurtful remarks. My parents did not know what to say and the doctors didn't know what to do. They admitted openly that they didn't understand what was causing it, only that it was an auto-immune disease.

To this day, I don't know how I got through the first few years of losing all my hair. I tried more medical treatments with irritants which produced a bit of hair but this fell out immediately once the treatment was stopped. The doctor explained to me that the risk of infertility as a side-effect of the irritants was too great to warrant further treatment. It later turned out that I was indeed unable to conceive, which was possibly a side-effect of that treatment.

I had tried every medical treatment that was available at the time, none of which worked, but all of which had major negative side-effects. For the next 30 years I was to try to recover from the medically induced health problems I had developed.

I learnt to cope with my condition but was always hoping that I could find a natural method that would work as I was no longer willing to accept all the side-effects that accompanied conventional treatments.

While I was training to become a health kinesiologist, a friend of mine who was also on the course worked on me to see if my hair growth could be restored. Using my arm muscle as biofeedback, she found out what it was my body needed to rebalance itself and to become healthy again. Holding acupuncture points, applying magnets to various parts of the body and a number of other interventions were aimed at sorting out those health issues that had made my hair fall out in the first place. After 16 sessions, I noticed that something was happening on my head. I looked at my scalp and found that tiny hairs had started to grow. It was the happiest day of my life and for weeks, I spent hours in front of the mirror just to see whether it was all still there!

Since that time, I have spent endless hours researching alopecia and have been able to help numerous clients regrow their hair. The stories I hear from them when they first come to see me are always the same, whether they are men or women – they are devastated and their confidence is destroyed. The doctors they go to see often tell them that there is no hope and that they need to learn to live with it. After all, it is not a life-threatening disease...

Alopecia might not be life-threatening, but its emotional impact is devastating. It can totally destroy your confidence and self-esteem, no matter whether you are a man or a woman.

Hair loss is now on the increase. Younger and younger women and men develop the condition where their hair starts thinning considerably or falls out in clumps. The medical profession has hardly moved on since I myself first developed the condition over 30 years ago – they still don't know what's causing it, and their standard fare is to prescribe steroids or chemicals which are applied topically. If they work, and they often don't, they have to be applied constantly. They also have considerable side-effects. Among those side-effects are that hair falls out even more rapidly. Chemical drugs can severely compromise the body's equilibrium. And for people who have lost all their hair on their entire body, even those chemicals are not really considered an option to help regrow their hair.

Regrowing Hair Naturally is based on my personal experience as well as on my years with clients who came to me to seek help for hair loss at my Harley Street and Surrey practices and who have been successfully treated with the methods described in this book. Most of these clients had been through the gamut of everything that is currently available in orthodox medicine. Quite a few of them had been told that their problem would go away by itself but then found it didn't. Some of them had experienced hair loss as a consequence of medication they were prescribed for another health problem. These clients were understandably reluctant to subject their bodies to more pharmaceuticals and medical drugs. All of them wanted their hair back without jeopardising their overall health. *Regrowing Hair Naturally* shows you how they succeeded.

In Part I of the book, you will find an introduction into the basics of hair growth and the various stages that healthy hair goes through in the course of its life. You will also find clear explanations about how hair loss can occur, and I promise you that there are several causes for hair loss that you have not read about in any other book! *Regrowing Hair Naturally* describes in everyday language how body systems can be affected by toxins, psychological stresses, nutritional problems and structural misalignments, leading to hair loss.

But first and foremost, this book is a practical guide to help you help yourself regrow your hair. In Part II, I will introduce you to ways of detoxing your scalp, regaining hormonal balance without drugs and using your subconscious mind to combat stress and promote hair growth. In addition you will find a list of vitamins, minerals and herbal remedies that can re-supply the body with missing nutrients and help restore hair growth. The book also gives clear guidelines as to which medical tests you should ask for when you see your doctor or dermatologist and how to interpret the results.

Regrowing Hair Naturally tackles the problem of hair loss from both the psychological and the physical angle, providing you with a great number of solutions that you can carry out yourself, as well as a number of therapies which can help detox the body and re-establish balance in your body so that your hair can stop falling out and regrow.

None of the solutions offered in this book are a quick fix. If you're lucky, your hair will regrow in a few weeks' time, but on average, regrowth takes months rather than weeks, so you'll have to be focussed and strong to see it through. Hair falls out quickly but takes a long time to regrow.

The good news is that you can regrow your hair, and you can achieve this without poisoning your body with chemicals and artificial hormones and all their side-effects.

This book will show you how natural remedies and treatments can help put your body back in balance so it can heal itself.

PART I

UNDERSTANDING
YOUR HAIR

CHAPTER 1

SOME BASICS ABOUT HAIR GROWTH AND HAIR LOSS

Some basics about hair and skin

I would like to start by giving you some information about how hair grows so that you have at least a basic concept of hair growth and the hair growth cycle. This will help you understand the causes of hair loss better, and it will also make it easier for you to visualise the images in the self-hypnosis exercise which you will find in Part II of the book.

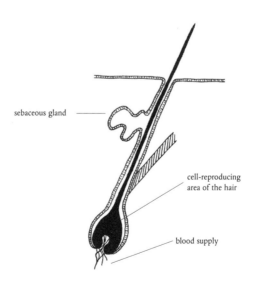

Figure 1 Sebaceous gland

The average adult has over 9000 square centimetres of skin surface. Depending on the body part, 1 square centimetre of skin contains about 10 hair follicles and 15 sebaceous glands, 100 sweat glands, half a metre of blood vessels, 2 metres of nerves with 3000 sensory cells at the ends of nerve fibres and a multitude of nerve endings and sensory receptors that record pain, cold and heat. The skin is crucial to the survival of a human being; that is why it is so dangerous if large areas of your skin are burnt – your body dries up and can no longer function.

The skin has a number of functions.

- It acts as a flexible physical support and cover for underlying tissues.

- It helps to maintain a steady body temperature through its extensive blood supply and sweat glands.

- It facilitates waste removal from the body via the sweat glands.

- It helps produce vitamin D.

- It helps keep the inside of the body moist.

The key role of hair in this context is to provide protection against heat loss. Hair keeps the head warm by trapping air near the skin surface to provide an invisible, insulating layer.

Hair is composed of a strong structural protein called keratin. This is the same kind of protein that makes up the nails and the outer layer of skin. Each strand of hair consists of three layers. The innermost layer is called the medulla and is only present in large thick hairs. The middle layer is known as the cortex. The cortex provides strength and both the colour and texture of the hair. The outermost layer is known as the cuticle. The cuticle is thin and colourless and serves as a protector of the cortex.

Hair grows out of a hair follicle. The follicle is an indentation of the outer layer of the scalp. The base of the follicle is shaped like a bulb, and at the bottom of this bulb is the dermal papilla. The dermal papilla is the crucial source of nourishment for the entire follicular structure. It derives its nourishment from a network of blood vessels in a deeper layer of the scalp.

Within the follicle are active cells which multiply and move forward to form a column of tightly packed cells, and it is these tightly packed cells that we call hair.

You can imagine that it is very important for the dermal papilla to get good quality blood from the surrounding blood vessels, because it is the blood that carries nutrients to the hair follicles.

The equation is simple:

- no blood supply – no hair growth.

- insufficient nutrients in the blood supply – insufficient hair growth.

- toxins in the blood supply – hair falls out.

Under normal circumstances, hair growth in each follicle occurs in a cycle which is divided into three stages:

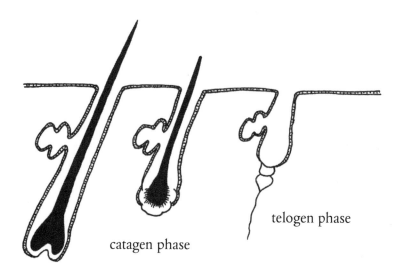

telogen phase

catagen phase

anagen phase

Figure 2 Stages of hair growth

Anagen phase

This is the growing stage of hair. During this stage, hair development is active and hair fibre is produced. This active growing phase of a healthy hair can be anything between two and ten years and is the longest phase out of all three phases. On a healthy scalp, about 90 per cent of hair follicles are in the anagen phase at any given time.

Catagen phase

This is the transitory stage between anagen and telogen. During this phase, the hair follicle regresses which means that the bulb-shaped indent in the skin begins to get smaller and rises up in the scalp. The dermal papilla now separates and withdraws from the inside of the hair follicle. The hair is still attached to the follicle wall but receives only little nourishment and the lower half of the papilla degenerates. This transitory stage lasts about 14 to 21 days.

Telogen phase

This is the resting state. The cells of the dermal papilla have now become inactive and the hair fibre and root sheaths stop growing so that the hair comes out easily while brushing or washing it. The length of this stage varies from person to person. In some people, the telogen stage does not occur as a new hair grows immediately. On a scalp with healthy hair growth, about 10 per cent of hair will be in the telogen phase at any given time.

Different types of hair loss

There are different types of hair loss, the three most common of which are alopecia areata, alopecia androgenetica and telogen effluvium. None of these conditions has to be permanent. Hair can regrow if you can find out why it fell out in the first place and then treat the underlying cause in a way that does not compromise the body's normal functioning. You may have lost the hair on your head only, but that doesn't necessarily mean that treating the scalp will resolve the problem. Hair loss needs to be tackled systemically, and understanding what has caused your hair to shed over and above the normal 70 to 100 hairs a day is a first step to finding a remedy.

Alopecia areata

The word alopecia was first used by Hippocrates and means 'fox mange'; the word areata means round. Alopecia areata is a non-scarring, inflammatory form of hair loss and occurs in men, women and children.

At the moment, the most commonly offered explanation for the occurrence of this hair problem is that it is an auto-immune disease, although neither doctors nor dermatologists nor trichologists (hair specialists) know why it is happening. Luckily you bought this book where you will find some explanations!

In an auto-immune disease, the body's immune system becomes overactive and starts attacking its own tissues. In the case of alopecia areata, the tissues that are being targeted are the hair follicles. Some people who suffer from alopecia areata also have problems with their nails which are made from the same material as hair – keratin.

Alopecia areata usually starts with one small round patch where hair falls out. This can happen overnight. The bald patch mostly shows itself on the head, but it can also occur in a man's beard or anywhere else on a person's body where hair grows.

This bald patch can stay the same size and then gradually begin to grow hair again, or it can become bigger, with more bald patches turning up. A sign that this type of alopecia is active and expanding are the so-called 'exclamation marks' on the borders of the bald patch. Exclamation marks are hairs that look like they have broken off.

In about 30 per cent of cases, the bald patches become worse to such an extent that all the hair on the head falls out. This condition is called alopecia totalis. If all the hair on the head as well as all other body hair falls out, the condition is called alopecia universalis.

A particular form of alopecia areata is ophiasic alopecia. The word ophiasic comes from the Greek word ophis for snake and means 'serpentine' or snake-like. In the context of hair loss, this means that the hair loss pattern occurs around the head horizontally, that is, hair falls out in patches along the front hairline, above the ears and along the base of the hairline along the neck region, so that only the hair on top of the head is left. This is a form of alopecia which is particularly difficult to treat, but it can be done, although it will take a long time.

Alopecia areata can also occur only in eyebrows, eyelashes or a man's beard. The received opinion is that in these case, the alopecia is usually confined to that area and doesn't spread to the scalp. However, I have seen a couple of cases where it did, so I would urge you to react promptly once you find any bald areas in your eyebrows, eyelashes or in your beard. The quickest way of finding out what is causing the patches is to see a kinesiologist or to have a hair sample test done.

Alopecia areata can last for many years. With some people, hair regrows in one place only to fall out in another. In some people, the hair all grows back only to fall out again in round patches a few months or years later.

When hair grows back, it usually does so as vellus hair which is very fine and without colour. Normal colour and texture only begin to develop later on. Some people experience changes in their hair colour during or after an episode of hair loss and sometimes these colour changes can be permanent.

The clearest way of identifying alopecia areata is to take a small scalp sample for microscopic examination. If the dermatologist finds that there is inflammation of the hair follicles, he or she can diagnose the condition as alopecia areata. I personally don't think this procedure is necessary. If hair comes out in round patches which have exclamation mark-shaped broken hairs along the borders, you can be sure that you have alopecia areata.

In my experience, any form of alopecia areata, no matter whether it is just one patch or the loss of all the hair on head and body, is a sign of heavy toxicity in the body. Detox has to happen slowly and with great support of the kidneys, adrenals and the liver. Health kinesiology treatment and nutrient support has to be tailor-made to the individual. Toxins have to be identified and removed with natural supplements so that eventually, the body can recover and grow hair again on a permanent base. A HGUK hair sample test can help establish the underlying toxicity that is causing the hair loss and determine exactly which supplements are necessary to remove the toxins.

Alopecia androgenetica

This type of hair loss is also called 'male pattern hair loss'. It shows itself in men as gradually receding temples and thinning of the hair on the crown. Depending on the individual man's disposition, the thinning temple hair recedes all the way to the crown and the hair on top of the head recedes all the way down to the back of the head, leaving a horseshoe-shaped fringe around the back of the head.

In women, alopecia androgenetica commences either by thinning hair in the crown area, sometimes by receding temples or a widening gap where you part your hair which slowly spreads over the top of the head. In women, there is usually no total hair loss on the crown area. Instead, hair grows only very finely so that the scalp can be seen through the hair.

In both men and women, this condition is thought to be caused by genetic factors and/or hormonal imbalance, and conventional treatment will deal with these two factors, using chemical substances in the form of tablets and lotions to reset the faulty genes and/or hormones.

Having worked over the last 12 years with clients who have this form of hair loss, I found that the true cause of androgenetic alopecia is not genetic. If it were, how come natural supplements are able to help the hair regrow? When I check a client's hair sample, whether it be a man or a woman, I invariably find toxins of one kind or another. Very often these are toxic metals, invasive organisms such as fungi and parasites, and/or food intolerances that prevent the body from functioning properly. Once these issues have been addressed with natural remedies, hair can start to regrow in many cases. This means that the hair loss was *not* due to a faulty gene but was only a symptom of toxicity in the body.

Telogen effluvium

As you already know, telogen is the phase in the hair cycle where hair becomes loose in the hair follicle and is shed easily during washing or combing. The word effluvium means 'flow out' and is used here in the sense of 'shedding'. Telogen effluvium is different from alopecia androgenetica in that hair is shed evenly over the whole head and sometimes also over other parts of the body.

Normally, only about 10 per cent of hair is in the telogen stage at any one time whereas most of the hair is in the growing stage. Clearly, if there is a higher percentage of hair falling out compared to hair growing, this will make your head of hair look thin and unattractive. We speak of telogen effluvium if a significantly increased percentage of hair follicles are in a resting phase than would normally be expected.

In some people, anagen effluvium develops as well as or instead of telogen effluvium. Anagen effluvium means that the hair is falling out during its growing phase. This is most commonly observed during chemotherapy or radiation therapy for cancer, but it also occurs as a result of poisoning with arsenic or thallium salts for example. Arsenic is contained in fungicides, cattle and sheep dips, paints and pigments and wood preservatives. Thallium is contained in, among other things, optical lenses, jewellery, dyes and recreational drugs.

Telogen or anagen effluvium usually first show themselves several months after a trigger factor has occurred. The trigger factor can consist of physical or emotional stress or hormonal imbalances.

Just as with androgenetic alopecia, I find that toxins are often at the bottom of this type of hair loss. This can easily be verified with a HGUK test with a hair sample. Toxic metals, invasive organisms and food intolerances, together with electro-magnetic field disturbances and some other factors, can cause the hair to change its growing cycle and prevent nutrient uptake into the hair roots.

Other forms of hair loss

There are two other forms of hair loss which are not due to illness but are self-inflicted.

Trichotillomania is an obsessive-compulsive disorder where a person pulls out hairs from their body. This can be either hair from the head, but also eyelashes, eyebrows, body hair or even pubic hair. If this hair plucking and pulling goes on over many years, the hair may not grow back again as the follicles are too damaged.

This problem occurs mainly in women and is strongly associated with anxiety and stress disorders and these have to be dealt with first and foremost to deal with the problem. I have had very good results with hypnotherapy for clients with this particular problem.

The other self-inflicted condition is traction alopecia. Here, the hair is pulled into a very tight hairstyle, often severely scraped back from the front and tied at the back.

The hair loss occurs in those areas of the scalp where the hair is being pulled particularly harshly. In traction alopecia, the hair is virtually pulled out of the scalp. A simple remedy is to stop putting this strain on the hair follicles by changing the hairstyle.

Further information

HGUK hair sample testing
www.hairgrowthUK.net
Go to the 'Services' section and download an order form for the tests.
Alternatively, ring my practice on +44 (0)1252 501050 for an order form.

CHAPTER 2

CONVENTIONAL TREATMENTS AND SIDE-EFFECTS

Today, more and more people, both men and women, suffer from hair loss. Family doctors, dermatologists and trichologists are often unable to offer a solution, especially if their patients' hair problems are severe or if the hair loss has persisted over many years. Patients are often told that they have to learn to live with it.

If the alopecia is not too severe and some hair is still growing on the head, patients are often prescribed drugs or hormones. Although these work for some people, they do have negative side-effects and usually need to be taken for the rest of a person's life. For other people, these same drugs make their hair fall out even faster. In severe cases where all the hair on the head and body (alopecia universalis) is lost, the medical profession offers no solutions at all. And yet, even in these severe cases, hair can be helped to grow again by using natural means.

You may be offered the explanation that your hair loss is a hormonal problem or an auto-immune disease, but if you were bold enough to ask where these hormonal problems came from or why your body's immune system is going on the rampage and attacking your hair follicles, you wouldn't get an answer.

Before I explain about conventional treatment, please let me be very clear about two things straight away:

1. Conventional treatment does work for some people, but it does not work for everyone.

2. Alternative and holistic treatment does work for some people, but it does not work for everyone.

In other words, there is *no* treatment, orthodox or alternative, that works for everyone. If you are hoping for a quick fix and you want to go for conventional treatment despite its side-effects, then I can understand that. After all, I went down that route myself when I first developed alopecia areata over 30 years ago. I know what it feels like to be desperate.

Conventional treatment does help a percentage of people who have hair loss, and that is excellent. The reason why I decided to put together the information in this section is that I found doctors and dermatologists to be less than forthcoming (and often downright ignorant) when it came to talking about side-effects. I believe, though, that you are entitled to make an informed choice before you go ahead with putting some pretty hefty chemicals in or on your body.

Here now are the most commonly prescribed orthodox treatments.

Minoxidil (also known as Regaine and Rogaine)

This is a lotion which is applied to the scalp. It is available over the counter and on the internet.

Originally, minoxidil started as an anti-ulcer medication but it was found to be more useful for the heart due to its strong vasodilatory effects (making blood vessels wider), and so it ended up being used as treatment for high blood pressure. When patients took minoxidil, it was observed that they started showing increased hair growth.

Minoxidil has to be applied for at least three months before regrowth can be expected. Hair often starts falling out again once application is stopped.

It is not clear how minoxidil works. It gets the best results for people with light forms of alopecia androgenetica or alopecia areata where there are only a few patches. It does not work for severe cases of hair loss.

Side-effects of minoxidil

I gathered information about minoxidil side-effects over a period of 13 years. The following side-effects have been reported to me by clients who have been on minoxidil between two weeks and one year (also see information at www.hairlosshell.com/minoxidil-side-effects-for-women): The side-effects of minoxidil include:

- skin irritation and reddening of skin
- itchy scalp, dry scalp and/or dandruff
- inflammation/soreness of hair roots
- burning sensation of scalp
- dermatitis and/or acne
- headaches
- upset stomach
- breast tenderness
- chest pains
- racing heart and/or irregular heart beats
- sickness and/or vomiting
- hair growth on face, forehead and ears in women
- increase in body hair in women
- increased hair loss
- decreased libido
- weight gain
- swelling of face, hands, feet or lower legs.

The stronger the minoxidil solution the more likely you are to have any of the above side-effects. Minoxidil should not be used if you suffer from heart weakness or heart disease.

Propecia (or Proscar)

Both Propecia and Proscar are finasteride drugs which are freely available on the internet. Finasteride is used for treatment of the enlarged male prostate but was found to help hair growth in men who suffered from alopecia androgenetica. According to the manufacturers, both drugs are only suitable for men and should not be taken by women.

Propecia and Proscar need to be taken for several months before regrowth can be expected. If you discontinue the pills, you are likely to lose your hair again.

There is no objective clinical evidence to assess the success rate of these drugs.

The drugs work by stopping the conversion of testosterone to dihydrotestosterone (DHT) which causes hair loss.

Propecia and Proscar are comparatively new on the market, having only been approved in 1997, and the only studies available are those the manufacturers supply. It is therefore unlikely that the following list is comprehensive. There are no long-term studies concerning the safety of these two drugs.

Side-effects of Propecia

The company Merck, manufacturer of Propecia, reports the following potential side-effects of the drug on its website (www.propecia.com):

- decreased libido

- erectile dysfunction and/or impotence

- decreased semen volume

- potential abnormalities of the external genitalia of the male foetus when the drug is administered to a pregnant woman

- male breast cancer

- early male andropause

- shrunken penis/testicles

- Peyronie's disease (crooked penis)

- depression.

Dr. Michael S. Irwig from George Washington University has set up the website www.propeciahelp.com, providing studies and information about the persistent sexual, mental and physical side-effects of finasteride, Propecia and Proscar, which continue for years after discontinuing the drug. You will also find a forum and a section where you can report side-effects that you experienced after the use of this drug. A class action lawsuit has already been filed in Canada, and a mass tort lawsuit is currently being prepared in the USA.

Irritants

These are usually liquids that are painted on the head. They irritate the scalp which produces an allergy, and this in turn stops the immune system from attacking the hair follicles in cases of alopecia areata.

There are two major irritants that are used: diphencyprone (DCP)/ diphenylcyclopropenone and Primula obconica.

If the irritants work, regrowth occurs within four weeks, although regrowth is usually only patchy. This method seems to work for about one third of patients. Regrowth often stops once the application of irritants is discontinued.

Side-effects of irritants

The side-effects of irritants can include:

- very strong itching on treated areas
- flaking of scalp
- constant burning sensation on scalp
- swollen glands
- fever
- anaphylactic reaction with fainting
- vitiligo (depigmentation in patches of skin)
- eczema with blistering
- numbness
- infertility
- mutagenicity (alters genes).

Irritants should not be used if you are pregnant or if you are planning on becoming pregnant.

Steroids

Steroids can be given as tablets, they can be injected into the scalp or they can be applied to the scalp as a cream. Whether you are prescribed tablets, injections or creams, the effects are the same – the steroids will end up in your body as they are absorbed not just through the alimentary canal when you take the tablets, but also via the skin if you have injections or use them topically as a cream.

Steroids imitate the action of the adrenal glands. If you suffer from Addison's disease where the adrenals cannot produce their own cortisone any more, or when you are in the grip of an anaphylactic shock, steroids are life-savers. Steroids have anti-inflammatory and anti-allergic effects and basically suppress your body's immune system. This is why they are used for auto-immune diseases such as alopecia areata, Crohn's disease, diabetes mellitus, lupus (SLE), multiple sclerosis (MS), pemphigus, psoriasis, rheumatoid arthritis (RA) and others.

Once you are on steroids, it can become difficult to come off them. As the body is supplied with artificial cortisone, the adrenal glands often stop producing their own. If you are currently on steroids, they will have to be phased out very slowly to allow the body to get used to smaller amounts so it can produce its own. It can take up to two years until the body produces enough adrenal hormone to cope with everyday stresses.

However, it is not always possible to induce the adrenals to produce their own cortisone again once you have been on artificial steroids for a long time.

If the steroids work, you can expect regrowth of hair within approximately four weeks.

Side-effects of steroids

Please note: These side-effects can occur within only a few days of steroid use, even if the dosage is low and even if you are only using a steroid cream on your scalp (Stanbury and Graham 1998; www.nhs.co.uk/conditions/corticosteroids):

- weight gain

- high blood pressure

- diabetes
- brittle bones
- muscle weakness
- Cushing's disease (fat belly and face)
- muscle wasting
- hyperglycaemia
- water retention
- thinning skin and bruising
- stretchmarks
- insomnia
- mood swings
- manic depressive symptoms ('steroid psychosis')
- osteoporosis
- cataracts
- glaucoma
- menstrual problems
- impotence
- allergic shock thrush of the mouth
- diabetes
- pain in the legs and back
- depression
- angina
- hair loss.

In children, there is the possibility of all the above side-effects, but also:

- retarded growth
- delayed puberty

- adrenal suppression

- osteonecrosis (bones die off).

PUVA therapy

PUVA stands for psoralen (P) and long-wave ultraviolet radiation (UVA) and is normally used for patients with psoriasis or those with other skin disorders. It is time-consuming as you will have to go for several sessions every week for at least 20 weeks before you can expect results.

Patients have to take a sensitising drug (psoralens) before the sessions and, as skin is sensitive to sunshine for a day or so afterwards, they must be careful to keep out of direct sunlight for a short time.

The success rate is low. It is very likely that, if hair grows again, it is only patchy. Hair is likely to fall out again as soon as treatment stops. Out of 39 clients who came to see me for hair loss, only two reported having had very slight hair growth after PUVA treatment. The other 37 clients had had no hair growth as a result of PUVA. The two clients with minimal regrowth lost all their hair again as soon as the PUVA treatment stopped.

Side-effects of PUVA

Clients who came to consult me after having had PUVA treatment reported the following side-effects:

- burning sensation of skin

- blistering of skin

- nausea

- redness of skin

- itching/stinging sensation

- headaches

- dizziness

- dry skin and wrinkles

- discolouration of skin/freckles

- squamous cell skin cancer

- eye damage if not wearing goggles during treatment.

CHAPTER 3

WHAT TESTS YOU SHOULD ASK FOR

Even if all these side-effects have put you off conventional treatment, you may still want to see your doctor, dermatologist or trichologist to have some tests done.

Iron, zinc, folic acid and vitamin B12 are among the essential nutrients for healthy hair growth, as is an optimally functioning thyroid. Under or overfunction of the thyroid can lead to hair loss. I would also recommend you have your vitamin D levels checked as this vitamin is important for hair.

Thyroid test

The thyroid is a very important gland in the body. One of its main functions is to control the rate of metabolism. This means that the thyroid is involved in the control of the breakdown of complex substances such as foods in order to turn them into substances that the body can use as energy. A healthy metabolism will also ensure that waste matters are divided off from the usable substances so that the waste can be excreted.

The thyroid is a vital link in the endocrine system, and even a small decline in the output of thyroid hormone can have serious effects on the metabolism levels which means that the body is not receiving enough nutrients and energy levels fall. If the thyroid underperforms, we speak of hypothyroidism.

If, on the other hand, the thyroid gets too busy, it begins to over-perform and we speak of hyperthyroidism. This increases the metabolic rate and causes extreme nervousness and irritability, sweat and loss of weight in spite of voracious eating. Other symptoms are palpitations and muscle weakness. It is most common in women in early adult life. The condition often shows itself in protrusion of the eyeballs and an enlarged neck region.

Just like hypothyroidism, hyperthyroidism can cause hair loss. The conventional way of dealing with an overactive thyroid is to take drugs which reduce thyroid activity or to destroy part of the thyroid with radioactive iodine or surgery. As it is very difficult to assess how much of the thyroid will be destroyed or how much needs to be taken out to reduce its activity, I would urge you to look at other solutions first. Once part of your thyroid is destroyed, you can end up with an underactive thyroid and end up having to take drugs for the rest of your life to help your thyroid to function properly. Health kinesiology and homeopathy (see Chapter 7), among other therapies, can be very helpful to regulate the thyroid, and there are also very effective herbs which will help the thyroid go back to its normal functioning again.

In Part II of the book you will see how you can find out yourself whether your thyroid is underactive by taking a simple temperature test over a few days. Go to Remedy #4 in Chapter 6 in the book for full instructions.

Zinc test

Zinc has been shown to be a beneficial trace mineral in the treatment of both alopecia areata and alopecia androgenetica. You will find more information about zinc in the section on supplements in Chapter 6.

It is quite easy to test yourself whether you are short of zinc with a solution called Zincatest made by Lamberts or your local supplier. This is what you do to test whether you are deficient in zinc:

- Take the test at least one hour after food or drink.

- Add 5 ml of solution to a 60 ml glass of water and immediately swirl a small amount of the diluted mixture around in your mouth for about 10 seconds. You can then either swallow the mixture or spit it out.

- Check what taste you have in your mouth.

- If you taste nothing, you have a serious zinc deficiency.

- If you have a slightly dry, furry or even sweet taste in your mouth, you are low in zinc.

- If you have a definite taste in your mouth which intensifies with time, you have a reasonable level of zinc in your body, but still not enough.

- If you get a strong unpleasant taste in your mouth which you notice immediately, your zinc levels are fine.

You may still like to have your doctor check your zinc levels to see whereabouts in the normal range you are. The normal range for zinc is between 11 and 24 pmol/dl, but the minimum level for hair is at least 14. So don't be satisfied with the answer that your zinc levels are 'normal' – they may not be high enough for you, so do the Zincatest in any case.

Iron test

This is a very important test, especially if you eat little or no meat. Make sure that the test includes ferritin levels as this is not necessarily part of a haematology test. It is ferritin which controls hair cell and growth production. The normal range is between 37 and 168 mcg/dl. However, the reference range can vary from country to country. Your doctor will tell you that your levels are normal, but be aware that you need a level of at least 70 for healthy hair growth if you are of European origin, so if it is less than that, chances are that you have too little ferritin to promote hair growth.

Vitamin B12 test

Vitamin B12 is important for cell production, in particular red cell production. The normal reference range for this vitamin is between approximately 148 and 738 pmol/l. (Levels of vitamin B12 vary according to geographical region due to different genetic make-up, and different dietary and environmental factors. This reference range refers to Europeans. In other countries, the normal reference range will be different.)

If your vitamin B12 levels are OK, your reading should be at least in the middle of the reference table.

Folic acid test

Just like vitamin B12 and iron, folic acid can prevent or heal anaemia.

The normal reference range for this B vitamin is between 7 and 39 nml/l. (This reference range refers to Europeans. In other countries, the normal reference range will be different.)

Your reading for this vitamin should be at least in the middle of the reference table for healthy hair growth.

Vitamin D test

This vitamin can be synthesised in the body by the action of sunlight (UVB rays) on the skin. Blood levels of vitamin D are therefore naturally higher in summer and lower in winter. Foods containing vitamin D are oily fish, fish liver oils, liver, eggs and powdered milk. Vitamin D is important because it regulates the amount of calcium and phosphate in the body.

This vitamin also has an important action on skin health. A deficiency shows itself in lowered immunity with increased susceptibility to infections, poor growth and brittle bones.

Vegetarians are more likely to suffer from vitamin D deficiencies than people who eat meat or fish.

The normal reference range for vitamin D is between 30 and 74 ng/ml. (This reference range refers to Europeans. In other countries, the normal reference range will be different.)

Further information

Zincatest
Lamberts Healthcare Ltd.
Can be ordered via www.bodykind.com
+44 (0)1892 554314

CHAPTER 4

CAUSES OF HAIR LOSS

There are a great number of reasons why your hair can start falling out. In the following, I have listed triggers for hair loss in three categories – physical, emotional and others. As you read through all three lists, you may be able to relate to some of them immediately as a possible reason why your hair started falling out or why it is not growing properly. In other instances, pinpointing the underlying cause can be more complex as the body can show a delayed reaction to a noxious substance or traumatic event. It is also possible that your particular hair problem was triggered by a combination of causes.

The body is an extremely finely tuned mechanism. Every muscle, organ, gland and cell of the body works in direct conjunction with all the other muscles, organs, glands and cells. The body is far more sophisticated than even the most advanced computer.

All parts of the body work together, with hormones controlling the balanced functioning of the entire system. Any workings in one part of the body will have a direct knock-on effect on all the other parts.

The body and all the body processes are geared towards keeping an equilibrium. If you eat too little the body is low in energy, so it will start using up its fat reserves to provide the energy for optimum functioning. If you are getting too hot, the body starts cooling you down by producing sweat which evaporates on the skin's surface and so returns the body temperature to normal again. If you get very frightened, all the blood drains from your head and face (you go 'white as a sheet') to provide all the blood for the muscles of the lower body so that you have the energy to fight or flee. Once the frightening situation or thought is over, the adrenals send out cortisone to counteract the adrenalin and calm the body down again. If your blood sugar levels get too high because you have been eating large amounts of chocolates or sweets, the pancreas excretes insulin to counterbalance the influx of sugars.

Problems start occurring when this ability to adapt is overstretched. If you constantly eat too much sugar in your diet, your pancreas can no longer keep up the insulin supply and you become diabetic. If you are very stressed or afraid on a regular basis, the adrenals can no longer supply enough cortisone to calm the body down and the adrenals become depleted.

If the body's capacity of rebalancing itself is constantly or traumatically overstretched, it can no longer readjust itself and ends up remaining in a permanently imbalanced state. It is at this point that you start noticing symptoms of illness or disease.

Unfortunately, we often overlook or ignore the initial warning signals that the body sends out, and we tend only to take action when the symptoms become acute or slow us down so much that we can't function normally any more. Worse still, conventional medicine often treats the symptoms only by switching them off so that we no longer get the warning signals. Often, this makes matters worse. Not only has the underlying cause been ignored, but now we are also likely to have side-effects from the drugs so that the underlying cause for our initial symptom gets obscured even further.

Once the body is struggling or unable to return to its natural equilibrium, the immune system is compromised and bacteria, viruses, fungi and other parasites have easy access.

Hair loss problems, just like any other health problems, are a sign that the body's equilibrium has broken down. In order to help the body function properly once more, it is necessary to check very carefully what has disturbed the body's balance. This can be tricky because by the time your hair is starting to fall out, a lot has already gone wrong. The hair problem is usually only the tip of the iceberg.

Have a look through the following list to see whether any of the causes could apply to your case of hair loss.

Physical factors

Hereditary disease

In some families, hair loss occurs through a fault in the DNA. Among those hereditary diseases are trichothiodystrophy and Pollitt's syndrome, both of which are characterised by brittle hair. Another such condition is Marie Unna type hypotrichosis where the baby is born with sparse and fine hair or no hair at all. Later on, the hair becomes coarse, wiry and twisted, and later still falls out altogether.

There may not be a lot you can do about your hair if you suffer from the above conditions, but I would still recommend you go to see a health kinesiologist who may be able to help you improve the condition.

To learn more, see the section in Chapter 7 on health kinesiology.

Lack of vitamins and minerals

Among the most important substances that the body needs to grow healthy hair are zinc, iron, folic acid, biotin, vitamin B12 and sulphur to name just a few.

There are a number of reasons why the body can be drained of some or all of these substances. Think about whether you have been in any of the following situations recently:

- crash dieting

- pregnancy

- excess sugar intake

- dehydration through lack of water intake

- eating too much wheat (bread, pasta, cakes, etc.).

To find out more about eating right for hair growth, read 'Remedy #6: Sort out your diet' in Chapter 6.

Hormonal imbalance

Any stages in your life where hormones are changing in any way can adversely influence your hair. Among those life stages are:

- pregnancy

- childbirth

- menopause.

In addition, there are also certain illnesses that involve hormones other than the sex hormones which can lead to hair loss. Among them are:

- hypo-pituitarism (Simmond's disease, Sheehan's syndrome)

- thyroid gland defects

- under- or overactive thyroid

- Cushing's syndrome

- juvenile diabetes

- polycystic ovarian syndrome (PCOS).

To find out how natural remedies can rebalance hormones, read the section in Chapter 6 on supplements (Remedy #7).

Extreme blood loss

When you lose large amounts of blood during an accident or a major operation, hair follicles are starved of nutrients and reduce their activity.

Severe or chronic illness

Illnesses, especially those which involve high fevers, can have a detrimental effect on hair follicle activity.

Overactive immune system

The immune system can become over-stimulated by a number of different factors such as vaccinations, toxic tooth fillings or parasites. It is essential to find out what exactly it is that over-stimulates your immune system. A health kinesiologist can help discover the underlying cause.

To learn more, read the section in Chapter 7 on health kinesiology.

Parasites

Parasites don't just eat the food in your gut, including all the nutrients that your hair needs to grow; they also leave their faeces all over your body. This can eventually produce a severe allergy and lead to even more serious health problems than hair loss.

To learn more, read the section about getting rid of parasites in the next chapter.

Incorrect bite

If your jaws don't fit together properly or if your jaws are too narrow, this can affect not just your posture but also the functioning of your brain. An incorrect bite can lead to tension around shoulders, neck and back, and this in turn will not allow sufficient circulation to get to the brain or the scalp.

To learn more, read the section about dental orthopaedics in Chapter 7.

Emotional causes

Stress

Stress is a major factor in hair loss, and in some people, stress alone is the trigger for hair to fall out. As soon as the stress is gone, the hair grows again. It is essential that you learn to relax and deal in a more constructive way with your stress.

To learn more, read the section in Chapter 6 on self-hypnosis for relaxation and hair growth.

Emotional trauma and sudden shock

Sometimes, a one-off shock or trauma can initiate hair loss. One of my clients was sexually molested by her father, and shortly after this event, she developed alopecia areata. Once the event had been worked through with the help of hypnotherapy and her body was rebalanced with health kinesiology, her hair started growing again.

To learn more, read the section in Chapter 7 about hypnotherapy and the section in the same chapter on health kinesiology.

Other factors

Accidents or falls

If the body receives a severe blow, the electromagnetic field in and around the body can be disturbed, leading to hair loss. The former Olympic swimmer Duncan Goodhew reports that he lost all his hair after he had fallen off a tree in the school playground as a child.

To learn how the body's electromagnetic field can be readjusted, read the section on health kinesiology.

Operations and scars

During an operation, tissues are cut and then sewn together again. The resulting scar often cuts across a meridian in the body. This can lead to a disruption of energy flow to the associated organ, and this in turn leads to health problems.

To learn how the energy flow of a meridian can be re-established, read the section on health kinesiology.

Dental substances

Some dental substances which are used to repair teeth are not compatible with the body's smooth functioning, and some substances such as mercury in amalgam fillings are actually toxic and are known to lead to hair loss.

To learn more about this, read the section about toxic dental fillings in Chapter 5.

Vaccinations

Vaccinations and jabs can over-stimulate the immune system so that it goes into overdrive and starts attacking the body's own tissues, resulting in auto-immune diseases such as alopecia areata. In particular the mercury in vaccinations in the form of thimerosal can cause major health problems.

To learn how you can reverse the ill effects of vaccinations, read the sections about homeopathy and health kinesiology or have a HGUK hair sample test done at www.hairgrowthUK.net.

Prescribed medication and over-the-counter supplements

There are drugs and supplements which can result in you losing your hair. Among them are cholesterol-lowering drugs, anti-hypertensive drugs, anti-histamines, ulcer drugs, anti-coagulant drugs, anti-convulsant drugs, anti-thyroid drugs, beta blockers, high blood pressure tablets, arthritis drugs, tricyclic anti-depressants, the contraceptive pill, HRT, vitamin A, retinol.

You will need to come off these drugs to stop their detrimental effect on your hair. There are many safe alternative solutions to physical illness which can work with your body rather than against it. A health kinesiologist, homeopath or bioresonance practitioner will be able to find these alternatives.

Cancer treatments

Chemotherapy drugs such as cytostatic, alkylating and anti-metabolic drugs can make your hair fall out, as can x-rays and gamma rays used in scans and radiation treatments. Hair usually grows back after the treatment is finished. If you still have problems with your hair a year later, you might need to support your body with nutrients and more water.

To learn more, read the sections in Chapter 6: 'Hydrate your body' and 'Supplements that help hair growth'.

Smoking

Smoking poisons not just your lungs but your entire body. Research found that smoking is detrimental to hair growth, so the way forward here is to stop being a slave to those dried rolled-up leaves! A hypnotherapist may be able to help you kick the habit if you can't manage it yourself.

To learn more about how to stop, read the section on hypnotherapy.

Other poisoning

Thallium, arsenic, lead, gadolinium and bismuth are all substances which can lead to hair loss. These may be contained in some recreational drugs, in optical lenses, cosmetics, jewellery, dyes, old water pipes, leaded paint, improperly glazed pottery and some DIY and craft products.

To learn how to detox from common metals, read the section in Chapter 6 about detoxing.

Hair products and dyes

Most trichologists will assure you that it doesn't matter what you wash or condition your hair with and that hair products cannot do any harm to your hair. This is not so. Some hair dyes can cause cancer, and I have had clients who were allergic to a substance in their shampoo and started losing their hair as a direct consequence.

To learn which ingredients you need to avoid, read the section in Chapter 6: 'Stimulate and cleanse hair follicles'.

PART II

ENCOURAGING
HAIR REGROWTH

CHAPTER 5

WHAT YOU *MUST* DO

There are some checks that you must carry out if you are having problems with your hair, but neither your doctor nor dermatologist is likely ever to mention any of them to you. These tests, however, are crucial if you want your hair back.

Hair loss, whether it is alopecia areata, alopecia androgenetica or telogen effluvium, shows that your body is not working as it should. The main reason for an imbalanced system that I have found in my practice is that there is some form of toxicity in the body. Two of the most common toxicity factors that disturb hair growth are toxic metals and parasites.

The symptoms you are displaying may not give you a clue, and your doctor is unlikely to suspect these two sources of toxins – if you were to ask them whether they could check you out for these, your problem would probably be dismissed as ludicrous. Please don't give up, and don't let yourself be swayed from checking these factors.

In what follows, I give you very important information on how toxicity can not only negatively affect your hair growth but also your general health. You will have to take responsibility for your own well-being and act on the information – your doctor will in all probability not.

Make sure you go to someone who can assist you with finding out. It is unlikely that conventional medicine will offer you comprehensive tests concerning toxicity, so I have given you contact details of associations who will be able to assist you. This means that you will have to pay for the treatment privately, but it is essential you do this in order to help your hair regrow.

Remedy #1: Replace toxic dental fillings

Stand in front of a mirror and have a look in your mouth. Can you see any silver-grey fillings? If so, how many? Do you know whether you have any root canal fillings? Do you have any crowns that were fitted before 1980? This could mean that you have amalgam underneath the crowns. And even after that date, you may still have fillings containing mercury underneath your crowns, seeping poisons directly into your body.

If you have silver-grey fillings in your teeth, you may already have found the source of your hair loss problems. Over 50 per cent of silver dental fillings, also known as amalgam fillings, are made of mercury. Mercury is a powerful biological poison and extremely toxic. It is even more toxic than lead, cadmium and arsenic. When you chew, grind your teeth, brush your teeth or eat hot or acidic foods, mercury vapours are released from these fillings.

The British Dental Association insists that mercury is made harmless when combined with other metals, but as early as 1993, the US Public Health Service released a report that confirmed that small amounts of mercury vapour are released from mercury fillings and can be absorbed into the body (US Public Health Service 1993). However, it was claimed that these vapours only affected a small number of allergic individuals. But when the World Health Organization reviewed the scientific literature (1990, 2008), it found that the public's highest daily exposure to mercury comes from dental amalgam fillings. It determined that the daily retained intake of mercury is from 3 to 17 micrograms per day from dental fillings, compared with about 2.6 micrograms per day from fish and seafood, air and water pollution. The committee also concluded that there was no such thing as a 'safe' level of mercury exposure. This means that, however minuscule mercury vapour release is in your mouth, there will be negative consequences. There is no safe level of mercury.

In 1988, scrap dental amalgam was declared a hazardous waste by the Environmental Protection Agency (British Dental Association 2007; Health and Safety Executive 2002). Outside your mouth, scrap dental amalgam has to be stored in an unbreakable, tightly sealed container away from heat. It also has to be left untouched and stored under liquid glycerine. There is clearly a contradiction here: when dental amalgam is in your mouth, it is supposed to be harmless, but once it is out of your mouth, it is highly toxic? Bear this in mind if your dentist assures you that your amalgam fillings are perfectly safe!

Dentists who are handling mercury on a daily basis have the highest rates of suicide among professions as well as the highest utilisation rate of medical insurance according to the industry (McComb 1997; Sancho and Ruiz 2010). At the University of North Texas, it was found that 90 per cent of dentists had neuropsychological dysfunction (Ericson and Källen 1989; Rowland *et al.* 1994; Sikorski *et al.* 1986). Female dental personnel who are handling mercury have higher rates of spontaneous abortions, raised incidence of premature labour and elevated perinatal mortality when compared with females in other professions. Another study of dental personnel showed a high incidence of spina bifida births (Matte, Mulinare and Erickson). These studies all show a positive correlation between mercury levels, reproductive failure and menstrual cycle disorders.

Sources of mercury include:

- fungicides and pesticides
- cosmetics
- dental fillings (silver-grey amalgams)
- mercury handled by dentists/dental assistants
- seafood (tuna, swordfish)
- medicines
- laxatives
- inks used in printing and tattoos
- some types of paint
- refined grains and seeds
- chlorine bleaches
- contact lens solutions
- injectable vitamins and drugs
- felt

- fabric softener

- floor waxes and polishes

- film

- broken thermometers and barometers

- antiseptic creams and lotions

- nasal sprays

- vaccinations (thimerosal).

Over the years, I found that clients displaying the symptoms listed below recovered partially or completely from these symptoms when their amalgam fillings were removed and a mercury detox programme was carried out:

- fevers and chills

- fatigue and chronic fatigue

- headaches

- insomnia

- loss of sex drive

- depression

- numbness and tingling in hands and/or arms

- painful arms and legs

- irritability

- hair loss

- asthma

- MS (multiple sclerosis)

- epileptic fits

- learning difficulties

- irregular heart beat and racing heart

- chest pains

- immune suppression
- birth defects
- infertility
- kidney damage
- brain damage
- stomach damage
- liver damage
- nausea
- inflammation of the digestive tract
- abdominal cramps (IBS)
- diminished urine output
- excessive production of saliva
- loosening of teeth
- loss of appetite
- Alzheimer's
- anaemia anxiety
- sensitive tongue
- metallic taste in mouth
- receding gums
- allergies and skin rashes
- epileptic fits and seizures
- auto-immune diseases.

How mercury damages the body

Mercury is one of the sulfhydryl-reactive metals. This means that mercury will inactivate sulphur groups from biologically active proteins. Many of these proteins are enzymes, hormones or cell receptors, and their destruction causes havoc within the various body systems and throws them out of balance so that they cannot work efficiently any more. One of these systems is our energy-producing system; another one is our digestive system.

Mercury destroys the mucous membrane of the gastrointestinal tract which forms one of our most potent immune defences. Mercury is especially destructive against the kidneys, liver and the brain. Autopsy studies show a positive correlation between the number and size of amalgam fillings and mercury levels in the brain and kidneys (Björkman *et al.* 2007).

Mercury is also well-known for attacking the central nervous system by crossing the blood–brain barrier. Mercury toxicity can cause the same symptoms as MS (multiple sclerosis). Patients with MS have exhibited mercury levels up to eight times higher in their cerebrospinal fluids than that of healthy controls (Fulgenzi *et al.* 2012).

Mercury also crosses the placenta. When you have amalgam fillings in your teeth and become pregnant, you pass this toxic metal onto your baby in the womb. Even if this baby never has to have any fillings in their teeth later on in life, they can still eventually have health problems because of the mercury they got from you before birth.

Mercury and hair loss

Mercury has been shown to affect T-lymphocyte function (Ziemba *et al.* 2009; Summers *et al.* 2003). T-lymphocytes (T-cells) are part of the body's immune system defence army. Once amalgam fillings are removed, T-cells increase. When the mercury fillings are put back again, T-cells decrease again (Huggins 1993; Siblerud and Kienholz 1994).

There are three types of cells involved in the body's immune function:

- B-cells which engulf and destroy foreign cells.

- T-cells, also called 'helper cells'. Their job is to mark foreign substances that enter the body so the B-cells know which cells to attack.

- T-8 cells, also called 'suppressor cells'. They keep the B-cells from attacking normal body tissues, such as hair follicles.

Mercury destroys T-cells. When the ratio between T-cells and T-8 cells becomes disturbed, the B-cells start turning against the body's own tissues. This can lead to auto-immune disorders such as MS, diabetes, rheumatoid arthritis, lupus, alopecia areata and many more.

In 1992, a study found that nearly half of women with unexplained hair loss had increased mercury in their bodies. In two-thirds of the cases, the hair grew back once the fillings were removed (Labar 1992, cited in McTaggart 2005).

What you can do

If you have mercury fillings, the obvious thing to do is to have them removed and replaced with less noxious ones. I personally consider this an absolutely essential measure if you want to get your hair and your health back. However, it is very important to start detoxing before the fillings are taken out. The detox will then have to continue during amalgam replacement and for quite a long time after all the amalgams have come out.

If you have the amalgams changed without having detoxed beforehand, you can become quite ill. During amalgam removal, mercury vapours are set free which can cause further problems. This is why some dentists are reluctant to take out these fillings and will assure you that it is safer to leave them in. The truth is that it is not safe at all to have these fillings in your mouth.

When your amalgams are removed, your dentist should use a rubber dam in your mouth which is a piece of plastic that covers the inside of your mouth and only leaves free the tooth the dentist is working on. Ideally, your dentist should also have a suction unit which sucks the air away from your mouth and nose so that you do not breathe in the mercury vapours that are set free when the old amalgam fillings are drilled out.

Ask your dentist whether they are able to replace your amalgam fillings using the necessary safety measures. Be prepared to hear though that it is all nonsense and has nothing to do with any health issues you have. Many dentists are not aware of all the research on mercury toxicity that has been going on over the years. In that case, go somewhere else to have the job done. You will find contact details at the end of this chapter of an association of dentists who specialise in the safe replacement of amalgam fillings.

I would also urge you to make sure that your body gets the right detoxifying supplements before, during and after the replacement of mercury fillings to make sure that it can cope with the detoxifying process. Detoxification with supplements should also be carried out for several months after the amalgam fillings have been removed. For more information on supplements that help remove mercury from the body, see a health kinesiologist or have a hair/nail sample test done to find out which supplements you need to detox (see the further information section at the end of this chapter).

In the meantime, you can help your body start detoxing via the skin.

DETOXIFICATION BATHS

Take detox baths twice a week, with at least a couple of days in between each bath. Soak in a tub of comfortably warm water after adding 1/4 cup of baking soda (= bicarbonate of soda) to the water. Afterwards, take a warm shower and make sure you gently scrub down your skin on the entire body to help toxins be swept away from the surface of the skin.

Do this for two weeks. Apart from the two detox baths a week, you can continue bathing and showering as you would normally do.

After two weeks, put 1/4 cup of Epsom salts and 1/4 cup of baking soda into the bath water and continue to take these detox baths twice a week, with at least two days between baths. Again, make sure you take a warm shower afterwards, gently scrubbing the skin to ensure that the skin is free from toxins that have surfaced during the bath.

If you find that you get very tired after the combination of Epsom salts and baking soda, reduce the amount of Epsom salts you use.

Other sources of dental toxins

Even if you have no amalgam fillings in your mouth, it is worth your while to go to a holistic dentist and have them check on an x-ray whether there is any inflammation or decay in the areas of extracted teeth. When teeth are extracted, the remaining cavity can become toxic and cause severe health problems. Root canal work is another area where toxins can be released into the body. All of these problems in your mouth can affect your hair. Have it checked and sorted out or your hair may not regrow.

Besides mercury, the common metals palladium, chromium, nickel and gold can also cause health problems. All of them are used in dental work. A particularly grave problem occurs if you have both amalgam and gold fillings as they create electric currents in your mouth which interfere with the body's electromagnetic field (Johansson 1986a, 1986b; Walker 2003).

A health kinesiologist can ascertain whether your body is having a problem with any dental substances that are used in everyday dentistry and can also help your body rid itself of these toxins.

Further information

BOOKS

McTaggart, L. (ed.) (2005) *The WDDTY Dental Handbook*. London: The Wallace Press.

A comprehensive guide to the dangers of fillings, fluoride and other dental practices.

Available internationally from Amazon. In the UK, order directly from What Doctors Don't Tell You at www.wddty.co.uk, or ring their customer services on +44 (0)1371 851883.

This book will also give you lots of references to all the research that has been carried out concerning mercury toxicity.

Breiner, M.E. (1999) *Whole Body Dentistry. Fairfiled*. CT: Quantum Health Press.

An easy to read and very clear description of electrical and toxic problems caused by amalgams. Also a discussion about root canal fillings, the problems they can cause and safer alternatives.

WEBSITES

If you would like more information about the problems amalgam fillings can cause, please watch the following two films on the internet:

www.youtube.com/watch!v=XU8nSn5Ezd8
Shows film of how brain neurons degenerate upon exposure of mercury ions.

www.iaomt.org/videos (click on 'mercury' link)
Shows film of an extracted tooth with a 25-year-old amalgam filling that still releases mercury vapours when slightly touched with a rubber eraser.

Mercury-free dentistry

If your dentist cannot help, you can find a dentist who deals with mercury-free dentistry by contacting:

UK
British Society for Mercury Free Dentistry
www.mercuryfreedentistry.org.uk
+44 (0)1242 226918

USA
International Association of Mercury Safe Dentists (IAMFD)
www.hg-free.com
+1 800 335 7755 (US and Canada)
+1 707 829 7220 (outside US and Canada)
The website will give you mercury-free dentists in the USA, Canada and other countries.

TOXIC METALS CHECK
HGUK hair sample testing (see p.20)

Remedy #2: Get rid of parasites

Toxicity in the body is one of the fundamental problems in any illness. Sudden and severe hair loss is usually due to acute stress or toxicity which is poisoning the body. Chronic hair loss is often due to hormonal and nutritional factors or a slow chronic toxicity. Toxicity can cause hair loss because the toxins interfere with the nutrients and hormones that help hair grow. Some toxins interfere with the glands or organs that govern these hormones, and some toxins can even damage hair follicles.

In the previous chapter you read about amalgam fillings and how the body can become toxic through the gradual seeping of mercury from amalgam fillings into your body. Another way of becoming toxic is when your body is invaded by parasites.

Parasites are not confined to third world countries. Everyone is susceptible to them, men, women and children, rich or poor. It also doesn't matter whether you live in the countryside or in a city – parasites are everywhere, in the grass of your garden, your pets, the soil and the air. Here are some ways in which you can become infested:

- from petting or handling pets and not washing hands afterwards

- from contaminated water

- from contaminated food (particularly pork and shellfish)

- from eating rare meat

- from contact with grass and clay

- from mosquitos, fleas, tics and common flies

- from sexual contact

- from not washing your hands after having been to the toilet

- from another family member who is infected

- from contaminated air in an airplane.

Pets are usually infected with ascaris, a roundworm that can be easily transmitted to humans. It is therefore crucial that you:

- keep pets out of your bedroom

- *do not* kiss your pets

- give your pets a separate bowl for food and water

- *never* use family dishes to feed your pets off

- *never* wash your pets' bowls in the dishwasher

- de-worm your pets *at least* every two months with a herbal de-wormer

- wash your hands regularly with soap during the day if you frequently touch your pets

- wash your hands with soap after cleaning your pets' bowls.

Parasites affect your health by destroying body cells faster than they can be regenerated. This leads to holes in the tissues (leaky gut), ulceration and anaemia. Parasites also secrete toxic substances which can send your immune system into overdrive and produce allergic reactions, pain and inflammation. In addition, parasites can obstruct the intestines and the pancreas.

The symptoms of parasite infestation are numerous, but not everyone displays all of them.

One of the main signs of having a parasitic infestation is if you have an anal itch, rash or fissures (broken skin around the anus).

Symptoms will vary from person to person, and the following list is not comprehensive and may also indicate problems other than parasite infestation (see www.nvcentre.com/nvc2003/uni_symptoms_paras.php and www.humaworm.com/symptoms.html):

- chronic fatigue

- digestive disorders which won't go away

- constipation

- diarrhoea

- bloating and flatulence

- multiple allergies

- joint and muscle pains

- anaemia

- hives and rashes

- abdominal cramps

- eczema

- dermatitis

- itchy ears, nose, throat

- restlessness

- anxiety

- depression

- waking up in the night, particularly between 2 and 3 a.m.

- teeth grinding

- hair loss

- repeated infections and inflammations

- problems gaining or losing weight

- loss of appetite

- eating more than normal but still feeling hungry

- drooling while sleeping

- numb hands

- damp lips at night, dry lips during the day

- grinding teeth while asleep

- behavioural problems in children

- problems concentrating.

There are different classes of parasites and within each class are many different types.

Protozoa

These are one-celled and invisible to the eye. They can multiply very rapidly and take over the intestinal tract where they can cause pain, bloating, constipation and/or diarrhoea. From the intestinal tract, they go on to other organs and tissues.

Roundworms

These are visible to the eye and multiply by laying eggs. The eggs are sticky and may be carried to the mouth by unwashed hands or by food.

Flatworms

These are also known as flukes. They have complex lifecycles, involving multiple generations and hosts which can make it difficult to get rid of them.

Tapeworms

They are the largest intestinal inhabitants of man and they have a head that attaches to the intestinal wall of humans. As long as the head is attached, a new worm can grow from it.

The problem is that conventional laboratory testing can only detect some parasites, but not all. Radionic testing as carried out by kinesiologists and bioresonance practitioners, on the other hand, can show reliably which parasites are in your system and can also help the body get rid of them.

Candidiasis (yeast infection)

The same yeast that causes vaginal yeast infection can also cause hair loss. Candida albicans and other varieties of this fungus occur naturally in small quantities in the intestinal tract, but some factors can make this fungus get out of control and overgrow your bowels:

- the contraceptive pill

- antibiotics

- iron deficiency/anaemia

- diabetes

- steroid therapy pregnancy

- high sugar diet

- high carbohydrate diet

- alcohol

- stress.

Both candidiasis and parasites live in the intestines and eat the food you are ingesting. This means that your body is not getting the vitamins, minerals and proteins that it needs to grow hair, so it is absolutely vital to get rid of these uninvited guests.

Candidiasis can show itself as affecting skin and nails, or it can occur as a vaginal infection in women. In women who take the contraceptive pill, the candida fungus interferes with the hormonal balance. The pill raises the female body to a constant state of false pregnancy which affects the character of vaginal secretions and favours growth of fungi. Oestrogens in the contraceptive pill create a tissue climate that furthers candida growth, and this can also cause infertility.

Symptoms of candidiasis:

- nails showing white patches at the top of the fingernail

- vaginal itching, vaginal soreness

- white discharge from vagina

- painful urination

- recurring cystitis

- irritability

- premenstrual and menstrual tension

- anxiety

- heartburn

- sweet craving

- carbohydrate craving.

There are some very effective herbal treatments that can get parasites as well as candida out of your body to give your hormonal balance a chance to recover and grow hair again. For herbs that help, see the section on supplements in Chapter 6.

Giardiasis

This is a diarrhoeal illness condition caused by giardia lamblia (also known as giardia intestinalis) which is the most commonly reported protozoa worldwide. It is now estimated that one in six people in the UK are carriers of this parasite. Symptoms usually start appearing about one to two weeks after infection.

Giardia lamblia lives in the intestine of people and animals and is passed in the stool of an infected person or animal. The parasite is protected by an outer shell that allows it to survive outside the body for long periods of time. This parasite is also present in drinking water and swimming pools.

Ways to contract giardia lamblia:

- coming into contact with water that carries the parasite (swimming pools, jacuzzis, fountains, lakes, rivers, ponds, any water that is contaminated with sewage)

- eating uncooked foods which haven't been washed thoroughly

- accidentally swallowing the parasite picked up from contaminated surfaces (bathroom, babies' nappies).

Giardiasis is very contagious, so if you have been diagnosed as a carrier, you can easily spread it. You should therefore take the following precautions:

Wash your hands with soap and water thoroughly every time

- after using the toilet

- after changing your baby's nappies

- before eating

- before preparing food.

Avoid swimming in pools, hot tubs and jacuzzis while you have the infection and four weeks after your symptoms have stopped.

The tricky thing is that some people have no symptoms although they have the parasite in them. Generally, though, symptoms of giardiasis are:

- diarrhoea

- loose or watery stools

- stomach cramps

- upset stomach

- weight loss

- dehydration.

If your immune system is already compromised through toxic metals, invasive organisms, incorrect diet, vaccinations and jabs and/or pharmaceutical or recreational drugs, you are especially vulnerable to parasites. Parasites secrete toxic substances and thereby destroy body cells faster than they can be regenerated. Also, parasitic excretions tax the body's immune system and produce allergies and allergy-like reactions. Parasites can even stop vital organs such as the brain or the heart from working properly, so it is extremely important to tackle this problem if you want your hair back.

Further information

BOOKS

McTaggart, L. (ed.) (2002) *The WDDTY Guide to Good Digestion.* London: WDDTY Publication.

Order directly from What Doctors Don't Tell You at www.wddty.com or ring their customer services on +44 (0)1371 851883.

Available worldwide as an e-book from www.wddty.com/health-books.html

This book is an excellent concise guide to research into IBS, leaky gut, parasites, ulcers, coeliac disease and other digestive problems. It contains orthodox treatment information, homeopathic and herbal remedies.

WEBSITES

The following institutions give information about various parasitic infestations and how you can become infected:

UK

National Travel Help Network and Centre (NaTHNac)
www.nathnac.org/travel/factsheets/index.htm
+44 (0)20 3447 5943

USA

The Centers for Disease Control and Prevention (CDC)
www.cdc.gov/parasites
+1 800 232 4636

TESTING FOR PARASITES

HGUK hair sample testing (see p.20)

CHAPTER 6

WHAT ELSE YOU CAN DO

Remedy #3: Hydrate your body

Most of us have heard about those famous eight glasses of water we are supposed to drink every day, but few people really know why this is important. I would like to explain the reasons here because drinking water is one of the simplest ways of helping yourself to de-stress and rebalance the body's energy.

The human body consists of 25 per cent solid matter and 75 per cent water. Brain tissue is said to be composed of 85 per cent water. Every living cell requires water, just as it does nutrients and oxygen. In order to function properly, the body needs to be replenished with water throughout the day. The body functions because electrical impulses are sent through the network of nerve fibres which in turn trigger the activity of many organs and glands. In order to relay information efficiently, these electrical impulses need water as a conductor. Water also helps all the organs in the body work more efficiently by lubricating the digestive tract and detoxifying the body.

If you are dehydrated, all sorts of illnesses can follow. The kidneys start producing highly concentrated urine which can cause infections such as cystitis. It can also trigger kidney stones which form when the calcium in urine collects into small lumps. Drinking plenty of water keeps calcium dissolved, making stones less likely. Dehydration also leads to constipation as the soluble fibre in your diet cannot soak up water which would help it to be propelled more easily through the bowel. Constipation, in turn, leads to toxicity in the body.

When you don't drink enough, the body goes into an emergency state – it hangs on to any water that is still in the body. This is when we speak of 'water retention'. One reason for this can obviously be the overuse of salt, but if this is not the case, the only way to reverse water retention is to drink plenty of water. This 'reassures' the body that it is OK to let go of the stored water.

Emotional upset or physical exertion use up a lot of water in the body, simply because higher demands are made on our nerves. The body is in a state of high alert when we are under mental or emotional pressure or when we are physically very active, so that the nerves are working overtime, using up our water resources much faster than they would normally do. Unless you replenish this lost fluid, the brain cannot function properly. This is the reason why we get a headache and feel muddle-headed or confused when we are stressed. You may have seen how someone in shock is given a glass of water. This is an excellent first aid for someone who has just experienced trauma, as a shock will deplete the body in one fell swoop of most of its water.

Some of the following environmental and nutritional factors will also require you to drink more than just eight glasses of water because they dehydrate the body:

- eating foods that contain chemicals and additives

- eating processed foods

- living or working in a centrally heated environment

- living or working in an air-conditioned environment

- hot weather

- exercising

- drinking tea, coffee and/or alcohol.

Water cannot be replaced by juices or soft drinks. Even though they contain water, they also contain dehydrating agents.

Dr Batmanghelidj, an authority on water, recommends in his book *Your Body's Many Cries for Water* (2000) that you also add some salt to your diet. He points out that salt is an essential ingredient for the body, ranking in importance just behind oxygen and water. Twenty-seven per cent of the salt content of the body is stored in the bones as crystals, and salt crystals are part of what makes bone hard. This means that if salt has to be taken out of the bones in order to maintain vital normal salt levels in the blood, it will leave the bones weakened. Salt deficiency could therefore be involved in osteoporosis. Dr Batmanghelidj recommends approximately a quarter teaspoon of salt per day if you drink two litres of water in order to ensure a balanced intake. However, before you rush over to your salt cellar, please check how much salt you are taking in when you eat during the day. Many processed foods contain salt, and you may already be using that quarter teaspoon in what you are putting on your meals!

Water should be taken regularly throughout the day, whether you feel thirsty or not. When you are stressed, you need to drink even more than the usual eight glasses. It is best if the water is mouth-warm (rather than room temperature) as it is easier for the body to use the water if it is warm rather than cool. However, if you can't stand warm water, then drink cold water. It's better to drink cold water than no water at all.

Here are some tips on how to best drink water:

- Drink small amounts often rather than one whole glass in one go.

- If you are not used to drinking water, start with one glass a day and work your way up to eight glasses per day over the period of four weeks.

- If you don't like the taste of water, drink it with a straw.

- Still water is better than carbonated water.

- Avoid tap water. Get a charcoal water filter jug to take the chlorine out.

- Always carry a water bottle with you wherever you are so you can drink water regularly.

Important

Any supplements you are taking won't work unless you drink enough water! Without water, supplements cannot go into the cells and without water, toxins cannot be flushed out of the body.

What is the connection between dehydration and hair loss?

If you are losing hair, something is not working in your body. Toxins have an adverse effect on hormones because the liver and kidneys don't function as they should. Your body needs to have plenty of water to help detox the liver and kidneys so that your hormones can rebalance again.

Drinking plenty of good-quality water will not bring your hair back on its own. The body usually requires more help to get rid of toxins than just the water. But water will considerably improve the quality of your skin and promote the healing process that leads to new hair growth. So if you want your hair back sooner rather than later, drink your eight glasses of water and cut down on foods and drinks that dehydrate you.

Further information

BOOKS

Batmanghelidj, F. (2000) *Your Body's Many Cries For Water.* London, Sydney and Los Angeles, CA: Tagman Press.

Remedy #4: Check your thyroid

When you have been under stress for a long time, your glands will have taken the brunt of the onslaught. A gland is an organ that secretes hormones into the bloodstream and causes a physiological change. For example, thyroid, adrenals and thymus glands all have important and specific functions in maintaining health and well-being in the body. Organs such as the heart, liver and spleen can also be classified as glands, even though they do not secrete hormones.

In the past, our nutrition contained organ meats such as liver, kidneys and heart much more than it does now. Eating organ meats helped support the respective organ in the body. However, with recent crises in the meat industry, we have become very wary of eating any inner organs for fear of contracting BSE. Also, it is no longer 'fashionable' to eat animal organs and few restaurants have them on their menu now. However, when we are stressed out and running on empty, our glands need support.

One of these glands is the thyroid which sits like a bow tie around the front part of the neck. One of its main functions is to control the rate of metabolism. It is a vital link in the endocrine system, and even a small decline in the output of the thyroid hormone can have serious effects on metabolic levels. If the thyroid underperforms, we speak of hypothyroidism. If the thyroid is over-performing, the term used is hyperthyroidism. In either case, your hair growth can be negatively affected.

If your thyroid underperforms

There are many reasons why your thyroid could underperform. Here are some of them (Budd 2000):

- you are born with a defective thyroid
- you have been treated for hyperthyroidism with radioactive iodine or have had part of the thyroid removed
- you have taken drugs such as:
  - lithium (for psychiatric illnesses)
  - phenyl-butazone (for ankylosing spondylitis)
  - tolbutamide (for diabetes)
  - beta-blockers (for high blood pressure or anxiety)
  - salicylates (to treat pain)
  - androgens (male sex hormones)
  - sulphonamides (antibacterial)
  - chlorpromazine (tranquillisers)
  - phenytoin (for epilepsy)
  - carbamazepine (for epilepsy and trigeminal neuralgia)
  - levodopa (for Parkinson's disease)
- supplementing the diet with too much iodine, either with supplements or with iodine-rich food (e.g. seafood) so that the thyroid gives up producing its own iodine
- constant stress, shock or trauma

- toxicity through dental materials such as amalgam and root canal fillings (see previous chapter)

- candidiasis and other parasitic problems (see previous chapter)

- having had lots of dental work done and consequently developing a misalignment of the jaw which in turn results in disturbed thyroid function

- having any operations in the region of your neck, for example tonsillectomy

- whiplash injury

- menopause

- nutritional deficiencies.

If your thyroid is underperforming, you can develop the following symptoms:

- depression

- anxiety

- deteriorating memory

- hair loss

- weight gain

- loss of libido

- fatigue

- cold hands and feet.

A simple way of checking whether your thyroid needs support is to use the axillary temperature test. Do the following:

- Place a thermometer under the arm as soon as you wake up.

- Keep it in position for ten minutes before checking. (Traditional glass thermometers are more reliable than digital ones.)

- Do not talk or move until the test is completed.

- Try to do this at the same time each day.

- Test for four consecutive days.

- Men can check the temperature on any four days. For women who are menstruating, the temperature is best measured on days two, three, four and five of their period. Before puberty and after menopause, choose any days.

The normal temperature range is 97.8°F–98.2°F or 36.6°C–36.8°C. If your average temperature measurements are below the above figures and if you display any of the symptoms described above, you could be suffering from an underfunctioning thyroid.

If you want to have your thyroid function checked, you can have standard laboratory tests done through your doctor or, if you are willing to pay for it yourself, get the tests done privately as you will be given the results personally. Make sure that not only the free thyroxine (T4) levels are tested, but also the thyroid-stimulating hormone (TSH) levels. If T4 levels are at the lower end of the normal range and TSH levels at the higher end, this is an indication of reduced thyroid function, even though the laboratory may tell you that your thyroid function is 'normal'. However, please remember that even a slight underfunction of the thyroid can cause the above symptoms.

WHAT YOU CAN DO TO IMPROVE AN *UNDER*ACTIVE THYROID
1. Diet
Cut down on goitregens. These are foods that reduce the uptake of iodine by the thyroid:

- cabbage
- cauliflower
- kohlrabi
- sprouts
- kale
- swede
- turnip
- mustard
- soya
- sweetcorn

- millet

- peanuts

- pine nuts

- almonds

- walnuts.

2. Stress control

- Learn to relax by doing some meditation or yoga every day, even if it is only for ten minutes.

- If you feel that you cannot handle your stress on your own, learn self-hypnosis (see later in this chapter) or see a good hypnotherapist who can teach you how to relax body and mind.

- If you suffer from anxiety and depression, consider counselling, psychotherapy or analytical hypnotherapy to help you work through what happened in the past.

3. Testing for supplements

- Consult a health kinesiologist who can test which supplements you need to help your thyroid work more efficiently again.

- Have a HGUK hair sample analysis carried out to establish which supplements can help your thyroid.

If your thyroid overperforms

There is no test that you can carry out yourself as you can for an underactive thyroid. You will have probably already seen your doctor if you have had any of the symptoms of an overactive thyroid:

- nervousness

- irritability

- sweating

- loss of weight

- voracious appetite

- palpitations

- muscle weakness

- protrusion of eyeballs

- rapid pulse

- tremor of hands

- enlarged neck

- hair loss.

What your doctor will in all likelihood recommend is that you take drugs that reduce thyroid activity, or alternatively, that part of your thyroid is destroyed with radioactive iodine or removed with surgery. *Do not do any of these things.* Once you have had part of the thyroid destroyed, that's it. You can't get it back and it won't regrow. No doctor knows exactly how much they need to destroy or remove, and you will in all likelihood end up with an underactive thyroid. Remember that both an overactive and an underactive thyroid can cause hair loss.

Instead of any of the above radical treatments, consider finding out the reason for the overactivity. Something is aggravating your thyroid, and you need to know what it is. Have your teeth checked and see a health kinesiologist who has the necessary test kits to run different tests to see what is going wrong in your body. Have a HGUK hair or nail sample test done to see which supplements you need to help the thyroid function normally again.

Further information

BOOKS

Budd, M. (2000) *Why Am I So Tired? Is Your Thyroid Making You Ill?* London: Thorsons.
Peiffer, P. (2003) *Total Stress Relief.* London: Piatkus.
Peiffer, P. (1989) *Positive Thinking.* London: Thorsons.

USEFUL ADDRESSES

The Association for Professional Hypnosis and Psychotherapy (APHP)
www.aphp.co.uk
UK: +44 (0)1702 347691

USA: +1 612 251 6990

The APHP maintains directories of Certified Hypnotherapists (UK-based and worldwide), competent and properly trained therapists. All APHP members are required to continue ongoing training and supervision. Lists of approved practitioners and training schools can be found on the website.

Health Kinesiology UK
www.hk4health.co.uk
+44 (0)8707 655980

Metanoia Institute (person-centred counselling)
www.metanoia.ac.uk
+44 (0)20 8579 2505

The Peiffer Foundation (positive thinking counselling)
www.vera-peiffer.com
+44 (0)1252 501050

USA, Canada, New Zealand, Israel and Europe
www.subtlenergy.com
Canada: +1 705 696 3176

Supplement test
HGUK hair sample testing (see p.20)

Remedy #5: Self-hypnosis for relaxation and hair growth

In self-hypnosis, you become your own therapist and use the power of your subconscious mind to influence particular body processes. Self-hypnosis is ideal for helping yourself relax physically and mentally. In addition, it can have a very beneficial effect on activating the necessary body processes to start your hair growing again.

Hypnosis has a long history of helping with physical problems, from hayfever, asthma, eczema and sleeping problems to IBS, infertility and ulcers. It is still not fully understood how the subconscious mind can bring about these effects, but a great deal of clinical research shows convincing results in many cases.

If emotional problems are underlying your stress problems, it may be necessary for you to see a counsellor or hypnotherapist to discover and work through the originating cause of your stress. However, in many cases, using the following script for self-hypnosis can already bring good results.

It goes without saying that you still need to have toxins such as dental mercury fillings or parasites removed from your body, or the best self-hypnosis in the world will not make your hair grow back! So make sure your diet is on track, your teeth are in good shape and you drink enough water besides doing your self-hypnosis exercise.

The best way of listening to your CD is to have headphones on as this enhances the effect of the exercise.

Warning

Never use your CD while driving a car or operating machinery. As self-hypnosis can be extremely relaxing, you could have an accident if you are doing anything else while listening to the recording.

When you use self-hypnosis you do not have to go into a deep trance to get results. Even if you can get just a little bit relaxed and concentrated, you will be able to improve the state of your scalp to stimulate hair growth. You should use your self-hypnosis script regularly for a minimum of six weeks, once a day.

Getting ready to listen to your CD

Make sure you won't be disturbed for a little while.

- Turn the answering machine on and the ringer of your phone off.

- Have a glass of water before you start. Drink it slowly.

- If you need to pass water, go before you start listening to your CD.

- Find somewhere comfortable to sit or lie down.

Self-hypnosis script for hair growth

Let your eyes close and take the time to listen to any sounds around you, inside and outside your room.

While you are listening to all these sounds, at the same time, you can also be aware of how you are sitting in your chair or lying on your bed.

Be aware of where your head is, your shoulders, arms and hands, the trunk of your body, your legs and your feet.

Keep your attention on your feet now and vaguely picture the muscles in your feet.

Gently tense those muscles and picture them shortening and tightening. Hold the tension…and now begin to relax them slowly, and watch in your mind as the muscles loosen, lengthen and smooth out.

Now gently tighten the calf muscles, from behind the knee down to the ankle.

Imagine the bundles of muscle fibres contracting and tightening. Hold the tension for a moment…and now soften those muscles.

Again, relax them and watch them lengthening and smoothing out… Now gently tense your thighs and your buttocks.

Hold the tension for a moment…and now begin to relax them until they are totally smooth and comfortable and picture them smoothing out and relaxing…

Be aware of how your legs are beginning to feel heavier and more comfortable…

And now move up to your belly area and your lower back muscles. Gently pull them together, tuck in your belly, hold the tension… and now begin to relax those muscles and picture them as they are lengthening and sliding easily back into their resting position…

And notice how your breathing is changing a little bit as those muscles relax…

Now move up to your chest and upper back muscles. Tighten them now gently, picture them tightening…and now let them relax again, letting them soften and expand and extend, and as your spine relaxes, you can let your back muscles get really comfortable and relaxed…

And now your hands and arms together. Gather your fingers into a fist, tighten the arm muscles, watch the muscles bunch up and harden…and now relax them again, letting the arm muscles relax and smooth out, elbows and wrists nice and floppy, hands and fingers comfortable.

And be aware of the heaviness of your arms…

And now your shoulders, neck and facial muscles. Hunch your shoulders up towards your ears, bite your teeth together, frown… and now let them go again, letting the shoulders sink down and down and allow your jaw muscles to loosen up comfortably – just relaxing...

And as you feel your body begin to relax, focus your attention on your back and feel the warmth in your back...

And as you become aware of the warmth in your back, keep your body very still and keep your head very still and open your eyes and look at a spot on the ceiling. Keep your eyes firmly fixed on that spot, don't let your eyes wander away, keep them firmly fixed on that one spot, and as you do, you notice your eyelids getting heavier and wanting to close, but try to keep them open and keep them fixed on that spot on the ceiling a little longer, even though your eyelids begin to get really heavy now, and it would be so much easier to let them close, but persist a little longer, keeping that spot on the ceiling firmly in your vision, even though your vision is beginning to blur a little and to fade in and out of focus, and as the spot on the ceiling becomes a bit hazy and you have to blink more often, your lids become so heavy that it is easier to let them close and to keep them closed, so allow them to close now, easily and effortlessly allowing the eyelids to close and rest...

And now imagine that you are standing at the top of a beautiful staircase which leads down into self-hypnosis, leading down to a white door with a golden handle.

In a moment, I'm going to count down from 10 to 0, and as I'm counting, I'd like you to walk down the steps of the self-hypnosis staircase, walking down into deeper and more comfortable relaxation.

10–9–8–7–6–5–4–3–2–1–0.

And now you find yourself in front of the white door, and on the door is a sign that says Self-Hypnosis Room. Reach out your hand, turn the golden handle and open the door just a little, so you can peep through the doorway. And you see that there is a lovely room behind the door, so you might as well open the door a little bit more and step through the doorway into the room and close the door behind you.

Now you find yourself in a room that is furnished just as you would like your very own private room to be furnished, with all your favourite bits and pieces in it. Take a moment to look around and familiarise yourself with your room. Maybe you can see the room in great detail and maybe you can't, but it doesn't really matter. The only thing that is important is that you realise that this is your own private room. No-one has ever been in this room before, and no-one except yourself will ever go into this room, so it is really totally private.

This room is the still centre of your mind where everything is possible.

Somewhere in the room you will find a comfortable chair, and the chair is covered with thick soft cushions and blankets, and it looks so comfortable and inviting that you find yourself going over and sitting down in it. Let yourself sink back into the comfortable softness of the cushions and now you can really relax. Just now, nobody wants anything and nobody expects anything, and there is nothing left for you to do but drift along on that comfortable feeling of relaxation.

And because you feel comfortable and safe, you might as well let your eyes close, and with your eyes closed, you can still feel the peace and stillness of your room around you, soothing and relaxing you as you let the everyday world just drift away so that you are left calm and peaceful and relaxed.

And as you are continuing to drift deeper into comfortable self-hypnosis, you can also be aware of how powerful your subconscious mind is. Your subconscious mind is always working for you, day and night, night and day, shifting thoughts and ideas into the right place in your mind. But your subconscious mind can do even more – it can help improve your health, it can activate organs and glands, nerves and fibres and tissues and cells in the entire body. Your subconscious mind can switch off pain, it can generate energy and it can reactivate hair growth, provided it is given the right instructions.

And as you continue to relax even more deeply, you are in contact with your subconscious mind, giving it all the relevant instructions to reactivate hair growth. You are now giving it all the relevant instructions to reactivate hair growth.

The first instruction your subconscious needs is to flush out toxins from your body to clean your scalp thoroughly.

Think the words: *Flush out toxins. Flush out toxins.*

The glass of water you drank earlier has already started going around your system, beginning to flush out the inner organs so that your circulation can begin to carry off any toxins and debris away from the scalp and out of the rest of your body. Imagine a stream of bubbles going through your body, oxygenating and cleaning all the muscles and organs, all the tissues and cells. Imagine a stream of bubbles energising your entire body, as if you had little cleaning particles travelling through your entire system, your arms and legs, your chest and abdomen, your shoulders, neck and face and all the way up into your scalp, cleaning and flushing out any debris, any toxins, any obstructions to healthy hair growth.

These bubbling particles clean out all the muscles and organs, all the tissues and every single cell in your body, travelling all the way up to your scalp where they are flushing away any debris, any toxins, any blockages to the cells that generate hair from the hair follicles. And the bubbling particles carry the debris and the toxins and blockages away from your scalp, away from your scalp, leaving it clean and free so that all the pores can breathe, so that all the cells can function again.

Imagine a stream of clean, clear bubbles moving up through your body, carried by the water you drank earlier, and as these clean, clear bubbles are moving through your scalp, they take with them all the toxins, all the debris and all the obstructions and carry them away from the scalp and out of your body through the tips of your fingers and the tips of your toes, leaving your scalp clean and refreshed and every cell in your scalp clean and alive and functioning perfectly.

Imagine all the hair follicles clean and fresh, ready to start forming new hairs, ready to start becoming active again, to perform what they know perfectly well how to do – grow strong, healthy, vigorous hair.

The second instruction your subconscious needs is to re-activate the hair follicles. Think the words: *Activate hair follicles. Activate hair follicles.*

In order to help your hair follicles perform their task quickly and efficiently, go to the energy centre of your body, wherever you feel this is. You may think of it as being in your heart region, your stomach area or in any other part of your body. Just follow your intuition and locate that energy centre from which emanates all the strength in your body, all the energy, all the healing power.

Imagine a switch or button which works the energy levels for hair growth. Find that switch or button that relates to hair growth. If you can't see it in your mind's eye, imagine what it would look like if you could see it. Even if you only have a hazy idea of what the energy switch looks like, that's fine. Imagine yourself flicking this switch from its *off* position to *on, on, on,* and the moment you flick that switch, the moment you do this, energy starts radiating throughout your body, sending vibrating, pulsating energy all the way up to your scalp, filling every muscle and fibre and tissue and cell of your scalp with life-giving energy, activating all the hair follicles, flicking them into action. And there is a sensation of warmth and stirring and shifting and moving in your scalp, as if your scalp was starting to wake up. Your scalp is beginning to buzz and pulsate, and as the entire scalp area is waking up, freshly oxygenated energy pathways carry nutrients to the hair follicles, essential nutrients that are necessary to form strong, healthy and shiny new hair. All the cells in the hair follicles now have the energy to remember how to make strong, healthy and vigorously growing hair, easily and effortlessly reactivating healthy hair growth.

Feel the warmth and the vibrating feeling in your scalp, notice that bristling feeling on your head, bristling with all the new hair that is now starting to develop in the follicles, growing stronger with every day. Feel that warmth of increased circulation in your scalp, carrying essential nutrients into the hair follicles, nourishing them as they start growing strong, healthy and shiny new hair.

Feel that sense of inner happiness and confidence that is beginning to fill your entire being, looking forward to all this new hair developing and growing and bristling on your head, looking forward to enjoying a full head of hair again.

And all you need to do is to drink plenty of water every day so that your subconscious mind can carry out your instructions and detox your scalp so that the new energy you are sending up to your hair follicles can begin to work and produce new, healthy, shiny hair that grows vigorously.

And stay with all these positive feelings as you take your mind back into your room, back into your comfortable chair in your private room, just relaxing.

And take these positive feelings with you as you make your way back to the white door with the golden handle, leisurely ambling back to that white door with the golden handle, still aware of the bristling warm feeling on your head, and let yourself out and close the door behind you.

Now you find yourself at the bottom of the stairs that you came down earlier on. Walk up the steps again as I am counting up from 1 to 10, and when I get to the number 10, open your eyes again and bring those positive feelings and the vibrating sensations in your scalp with you, feeling confident and strong.

1–2–3–4–5–6–7–8–9–10.

Make sure you only listen to your CD while sitting or lying down. Under no circumstances should you listen while driving a car or working machinery. As there is a strong relaxing effect if you do the exercise correctly, you could easily cause an accident if you drove.

Further information

USEFUL ADDRESSES

The Association for Professional Hypnosis and Psychotherapy (APHP)
www.aphp.co.uk
UK: +44 (0)1702 347691
USA: +1 612 251 6990
The APHP maintains directories of Certified Hypnotherapists (UK-based and worldwide), competent and properly trained therapists. All APHP members are required to continue ongoing training and supervision. Lists of approved practitioners and training schools can be found on the website.

Remedy #6: Sort out your diet

You have already read about water and how important it is for health and hair growth. Now we will be looking at foods and how they can help or hinder healthy development of hair follicles.

Your body is a very complex and delicate system of checks and balances. Depending on what you are putting into your body, these checks and balances can work more or less efficiently. If you want your hair back, you are dependent on your body functioning at an optimum level. Only if everything inside you is running smoothly will the hair follicles get the blood supplies and the nutrients that they need in order to grow healthy and strong hair.

In this context it is important to understand that certain foods will actively discourage hair growth, and you need to know about them and avoid them as much as possible.

Acidic foods versus alkaline foods

In order to produce new hair growth, you need to eat considerably more alkaline foods than acidic ones. Alkaline foods are those that the body breaks down into alkali which means they are high in sodium and potassium. Acidic foods, on the other hand, produce acid when metabolised and contain sulphur, phosphoric acid and chlorine, all essential for efficient metabolism.

Both acidic and alkali-forming foods are important for good health. The trick is to have the right balance between the two. Our fast food culture drives us towards a more acidic balance, and this is bad for hair growth. Ideally, your diet should be more alkaline. Some nutritionists will tell you that the balance should be 80 per cent alkaline and 20 per cent acid-producing foods. I personally find that this balance can differ vastly from person to person. Some people need a lot more acid-producing foods than just 20 per cent, so even if you aim for 60 per cent alkaline and 40 per cent acidic, that is likely to be an improvement on how you are eating currently if your diet isn't very good.

Have a look at the following lists of foods and see where the majority of your staple foods are.

Alkali-forming foods include:

- almonds

- asparagus

- brazil nuts

- buckwheat

- cauliflower

- carrots

- chestnuts

- coconuts

- cream

- cucumber

- dates*

- dried beans

- figs*

- fruits (except prunes)

- herb teas

- lemons

- lettuce

- lima beans

- milk

- millet

- molasses

- parsnips

- dried peas

- potatoes

- radishes

- raisins*

- soya beans

- soya flour

- tomatoes (only fresh ones)

- turnips

- vegetables (green leafy)

- watercress

- yeast.

Please note: Any of the above alkaline-forming foods will form acids in your body if you are intolerant to them, so it is important to check that you tolerate them.

Foods marked with an asterisk * are very high in sugars if they are dried, and you should therefore only eat them occasionally and in small amounts. If you eat these fruits fresh rather than dried, they are less of a sugar burden to the body.

Neutral foods include:

- butter

- milk

- vegetable oils.

Acid-forming foods include:

- breads
- cereals
- cheese
- chocolate
- cocoa
- coffee
- eggs
- fish
- flour
- grain products
- lentils
- meats (all)
- nuts (except almonds and brazil nuts)
- oats
- organ meats
- oysters
- pasta
- peanuts
- pearl barley
- prunes
- rhubarb
- rice
- sugar
- sweetcorn
- tea.

So if you have been living off burgers, pasta meals, sandwiches and teas and coffees up until now, you will have an over-acidic body, and you will have to make some changes to your diet if you want your hair back. Even if you cannot manage to achieve the optimal 80 per cent – 20 per cent balance, you need to strive for at least 60 per cent alkaline and 40 per cent acidic foods for a number of months to get any results.

Wheat, gluten and hair loss

You may have heard about a condition called coeliac disease. This is an auto-immune disease caused by an adverse immune reaction to gluten in your diet. Gluten is a mixture of proteins found in some cereals. The grain with the highest amount of gluten is wheat, but rye, barley and semolina also contain gluten. It is the gliadin component of gluten which is responsible for coeliac disease.

If you eat a lot of bread, pasta, pasties, cakes and biscuits and if you crave these foods, it is very likely that you have a wheat intolerance. The craving you experience is a withdrawal symptom which occurs if you haven't had the allergenic food for a while. Once you have eaten the allergenic food, you feel much better for a little while, but after an hour or so, your mood starts to deteriorate and you become irritable and cranky – until you have provided yourself with another 'hit' of that food. This vicious circle is also known as a 'masked food allergy'.

Gluten intolerance (coeliac disease) is not the same as wheat intolerance. I have seen clients who could not eat wheat products even when the gluten had been removed, so if you suspect that you have a problem with gluten or wheat, it is best to have it checked out with a simple hair or nail sample test. Many people who are intolerant to wheat are also intolerant to other grains.

If you are intolerant to *wheat* but *OK with gluten* you can have rice, millet, oats, rye, buckwheat, barley, amaranth, quinoa, sago and tapioca, *provided you are not intolerant to any of these.*

If you are intolerant to *wheat* but *OK with gluten* you *cannot* have sprouted wheat, spelt, kamut, cous cous, semolina or bulgur.

Important

If you are intolerant to *wheat* but *OK with gluten* you *cannot* have gluten-free wheat! You are intolerant to wheat, even if the gluten has been taken out of the wheat.

If you are intolerant to *wheat and gluten* you *cannot* have wheat, rye, oats or barley, but you can have rice, millet, buckwheat, amaranth and/or quinoa, *provided you are not intolerant to any of these*.

To find out whether you have a problem with wheat or gluten, check the following:

- Do you eat a lot of bread, pasta, cakes, biscuits or pasties?

- Does it improve your mood eating the above foods?

- Do you become irritable and restless a few hours after you have had the above foods?

- Does your irritability and restlessness abate immediately when you eat the above foods again?

- Do you feel bloated after having eaten the above foods?

If you answer yes to most or all of these questions, you have either a wheat or a gluten intolerance. This means that the continued eating of these foods will make your hair problems worse. If you are intolerant to gluten or wheat and if you do not strictly adhere to a gluten or wheat-free diet, there is a possibility that you develop an auto-immune disease such as alopecia areata or other hair loss problems such as diffuse hair loss.

If you do not tolerate gluten or wheat, your gut becomes inflamed, and this inhibits the absorption of nutrients from food which your hair follicles need to produce hair. This in turn will mess up your hormone production which can then cause problems with hair.

If you are gluten or wheat intolerant and have a hair problem, you will need to avoid eating these foods for quite a while before you can re-introduce them in small quantities into your diet without losing your hair again. A health kinesiologist can help you overcome the intolerance, but you will still have to avoid wheat and/or gluten for a while.

In the meantime, start reading labels. You'll be shocked to see how many foods have wheat in them. Sausages, baked beans, soups and most ready-made meals to name just a few. It is therefore important to read labels. Give your gut a chance to recover so it can absorb the necessary nutrients for healthy hair growth.

Sugar – enemy no. 1

Sugar is not good for you. Most people are aware of its detrimental effect on teeth, but the damage done by sugar goes even further.

White sugar is refined and stripped of all fibres, proteins and other nutrients. The remaining substance is then bleached, leaving only a single industrially processed chemical. Even if you don't take sugar in your tea or coffee, you are still being fed it in other ways as sugar is added to a great number of processed foods.

If you consume foods that contain sugar on a regular basis, you begin to do serious damage to your health. As sugar has small molecules, the body converts it very quickly so that it arrives in the bloodstream in less than an hour. This in turn floods the body with sugar which our metabolism cannot cope with. The pancreas now starts producing masses of insulin and as a result, only little sugar is stored – most of it is converted into fat and hardly any is available for energy. This translates into tiredness, irritability, dizziness and sometimes even fainting spells.

Too much sugar also leads to undernourishment of the body due to the leeching of vitamins and minerals from the body.

But if sugar is bad, artificial sweeteners are even worse, and there is extensive research to prove it. The most widely used sweetener is aspartame which is added to drinks and food as a sugar substitute. Aspartame is also in other sweeteners, so check the label of any 'diet' foods or drinks you buy!

Aspartame is actually an extremely toxic chemical. Although it is marketed as a diet product, it can cause weight gain because it makes you crave carbohydrates. But that is the least of your problems. Aspartame is a toxic chemical which can and does cause seizures (www.holisticmed.com/aspartame).

The reason why aspartame is extremely poisonous is that it contains wood alcohol which turns into formaldehyde once it exceeds 86 degrees (www.holisticmed.com/aspartame). Formaldehyde is grouped in the same class of poisons as cyanide and arsenic.

Aspartame attacks and destroys the nervous system, but it does so slowly as opposed to cyanide and arsenic.

Symptoms caused by aspartame poisoning are:

- spasms

- shooting pains

- numbness in legs

- cramps

- vertigo

- dizziness

- headaches

- tinnitus

- joint pain

- depression

- anxiety attacks

- slurred speech

- blurred vision

- memory loss.

All this could be diagnosed as stress symptoms or even fibromyalgia, when what it really is is aspartame poisoning.

Aspartame is the best documented artificial sugar which has detrimental effects on your health, but other artificial sugars are similarly noxious. Make it a rule to avoid *any* type of artificial sugar to be sure that you are not doing damage to yourself.

The moral of the story is: try to avoid sugar as far as possible and cut down drastically on your use of sugar in teas and coffees. Don't touch anything with a bargepole that says 'diet' on it, unless this refers to reduced fat.

Make it a habit to read labels and check them for any ingredients that are sugar, glucose, fructose or dextrose. Be particularly careful if a product says 'sugar free' – it usually means that sugar has been substituted with an artificial sweetener. Remember that the ingredients on the label are listed in order of greatest quantity, so if anything has sugar as the first ingredient, put it straight back onto the shelf!

WHAT IS THE CONNECTION BETWEEN SUGAR AND HAIR LOSS?

As you have seen in the explanation above, excessive sugar creates excessive insulin production. Insulin is a hormone, and we know that hair loss is, in many cases, connected to a hormonal imbalance. Hormones which are involved in hair loss are not just those connected with our reproductive organs (oestrogen and progesterone produced by the ovaries; testosterone produced by the testes); hair loss is also influenced by other hormones. A hormone is a chemical messenger which, having been formed in one organ or gland, is carried in the blood to another organ (target organ) where it influences activity, growth and nutrition of that organ.

Glands that excrete hormones are called endocrine glands. Among them are the pituitary gland, the thyroid and parathyroid glands, the adrenals, the islets of Langerhans in the pancreas, the thymus and the pineal gland. If you clog up your body with sugar or if you are constantly dehydrated, it will affect all these glands as well, and that means that they begin to overfunction or underfunction. This leads to further imbalances in your temperature control, your immune system and many other problems. If your weak point is your hair, this imbalance will then also end up affecting your hair growth cycle.

In the next chapter, we will be looking at supplements that are particularly helpful when you want to improve the quality of your hair or if you want to support new hair growth. Before you start using any supplements, though, make sure your bowels are in working order; otherwise, the supplements will go in the top and out the bottom without getting into your system. If your gut is not in working order, it won't be able to absorb the supplements.

The best way of helping your gut to work optimally to promote good nutrient uptake for your hair is with the following vegetable cleanser which will also be helpful against some microbes.

Cultured vegetables

You can use either one or a combination of the following vegetables: carrots, cauliflower, white, green or red cabbage, beetroot.

You can also put parsley (shredded) or garlic (crushed) into the mixture, but be aware that the garlic taste will be very strong even with only one clove. Also, *you'll* smell of garlic when you consume the cultured vegetables with garlic!

1. Buy two large preserve jars which have a rubber ring to seal them tightly.

2. Shred or grate one or several of the above vegetables into small pieces and fill both jars, leaving two fingers' width of space at the top.

3. Fill both jars with lukewarm water. Ideally, use filtered water or bottled still water which you have warmed up. Make sure all the vegetables are covered in water.

4. Break open two acidophilus capsules and empty them into one jar. Mix well with the water and vegetables. Do the same for the other jar.

5. Seal both jars and leave to stand on the kitchen surface for three days. Keep out of direct sunlight (you can put a kitchen towel over them). During these three days, the acidophilus bacteria can spread throughout the jars.

6. After three days, the cultured vegetables are ready to eat. Place both jars into the fridge.

7. Eat one tablespoon full of the cultured vegetables with every meal for at least two weeks before you start a detox with any supplements suggested in the next chapter.

Once you have started on a detox programme, use one tablespoon of the cultured vegetables with a meal, once a day for four weeks.

Further information

BOOKS

DesMaisons, K. (2000) *The Sugar Addict's Total Recovery Programme.* London: Schuster.

This is an excellent book with a very clever way to help you come off sugars and carbohydrates. Highly recommended!

WEBSITES
UK
Coeliac UK
www.coeliac.org.uk
+44 (0)845 305 2060

USA
Celiac.com
www.celiac.com

Remedy #7: Supplements that help hair growth

There are some basics that need to be right if you want to get your hair back, and these are listed here.

Remember, however, that even though you may supplement your diet with any or all of these minerals and vitamins, this is no guarantee that your hair will regrow unless you remove or deal with the cause of your hair loss problem!

I have not given you a recommended dosage for any of these supplements because there is no right dosage that suits everyone. It all depends on the state of each individual's health and therefore needs to be tested individually. At my practice, I have had clients who needed to take 100 mg of a vitamin per day, whereas another person needed ten times that amount. One client needed to take zinc for only four weeks, another client needed zinc for six months.

The HGUK hair sample test will tell you whether you need any of the following supplements and if so, how much and for how long.

Iron

Iron is a trace element and one of the most important minerals in the human body. Iron is important because it forms a constituent of the blood pigment haemoglobin which is contained in red blood cells and is the carrier of vital oxygen around the body. Iron is also found in muscles and is additionally helping in the release of energy in the body.

If there is a lack of iron, you can suffer from the following symptoms:

- anaemia

- fatigue

- light-headedness

- headaches

- insomnia

- palpitations

- weakness

- pale complexion

- itching.

Iron deficiency leads to hypothyroidism, which in turn causes an imbalance of other minerals such as zinc and copper. As a consequence, the body begins to absorb toxic metals such as lead in greater quantities.

People who are particularly prone to iron deficiency are women of childbearing age, women with strong menstrual blood flow, vegetarians, pregnant women, adolescents, athletes and the elderly. There are also a number of prescribed drugs which will cause reduced bioavailililty of iron. These are medicines such as tetracycline, penicillamine, levodopa, methyldopa and cardidopa.

Foods that bind with iron so that the mineral becomes unavailable to the body are bran and other high fibre foods, rhubarb, spinach and chocolate. (But then you don't eat chocolate any more because you read my advice about sugars, didn't you?)

To be absorbed well, iron should be taken in its ferrous form (rather than the ferric form which depletes vitamin E). Take iron together with vitamin C and vitamin B complex. Take iron with food.

Iron can cause damage to your health if taken in quantities larger than prescribed.

Zinc

Zinc has been shown to be a beneficial trace mineral in the treatment of both alopecia areata and alopecia androgenetica. Oral zinc has been shown to have an immuno-modulatory effect, which means that it balances out immune responses. As in alopecia areata, the immune system is in overdrive, zinc appears to help it calm down so it stops attacking the hair follicles. If, on the other hand, your immune system is sluggish, zinc will help it perform better.

Interestingly, zinc is required for the metabolism of thyroid-stimulating hormone (TSH), and if not enough zinc is available to the body, this can lead to hypothyroidism. Zinc is also an antagonist of heavy metals such as cadmium, lead and mercury and helps eliminate candida. In addition, zinc is also required for optimum balance of progesterone, oestrogen and testosterone and therefore also beneficial in cases where hair loss is due to hormonal imbalance.

There have also been studies which showed that zinc inhibits 5-alpha-reductase activity (Mervyn 1989) and it is therefore concluded that it is beneficial in diseases that involve an excess of dihydrotestosterone (DHT) which leads to alopecia androgenetica.

Signs of zinc deficiency include:

- eczema

- hair loss

- mental apathy

- lowered sperm count

- decreased growth rate

- post-natal depression

- loss of sense of taste

- loss of sense of smell

- white spots on nails

- susceptibility to infections.

You are likely to be low in zinc if you eat a high-fibre diet or processed foods with additives.

External application of zinc to the scalp can also be helpful in promoting hair growth as it appears that some people have zinc deficiencies in their skin despite the fact that they have normal levels within their bloodstream.

Zinc is an essential trace mineral and is best taken on an empty stomach. Some people feel slightly sick when taking it, but the nausea passes after a minute or so.

Vitamin C

Vitamin C is a water-soluble vitamin also known as ascorbic acid. It works as an anti-oxidant, maintains healthy collagen and provides resistance to infections. As you have already read in the section about iron, it also promotes iron absorption from food. Another important function of vitamin C is that it controls blood cholesterol levels and makes folic acid active. It produces anti-stress hormones and helps manufacture brain and nerve substances.

Symptoms of vitamin C deficiency are (Mervyn 1989):

- dry, rough or scaly skin
- broken thread veins in skin around hair follicles
- easy bruising
- poor wound healing
- scalp dryness
- brittle hair
- hair loss
- dry cracked lips
- inflamed bleeding gums
- loose teeth
- weakness.

You are likely to suffer from vitamin C deficiency if you smoke or suffer from diabetes mellitus, if you have just had an operation, take the contraceptive pill, antibiotics, barbiturates, corticosteroids, anti-arthritic drugs, if you are stressed, drink alcohol regularly, have an infectious disease or have gastric or duodenal ulcers.

The recommended daily dose for vitamin C is 60 mg, but this is far too little to give any results when taken in conjunction with hair loss problems. Any doses up to 3000 mg a day are perfectly safe, but not for everyone. Please bear in mind that everyone's body is unique and everybody's hair loss will have to be treated in accordance with the underlying symptoms and will therefore require a different dose of vitamin C.

If you would like to self-prescribe vitamin C, it won't be a problem if you take too much because the body simply throws out what it cannot use. A rule of thumb is that when you start getting diarrhoea, you are taking too much. Decrease the dosage by 500 mg and see what happens. If your loose bowels stop, you've got the right dosage. All you have to find out now is how long to take the vitamin C for. Always use a buffered vitamin C product which makes it less acidic.

You should not self-prescribe vitamin C if you have had kidney or gallstones in the past, if you suffer from haemochromatosis or have had renal failure.

Vitamin C is water-soluble and can be taken with or without food.

Vitamin B12

Vitamin B12 is also known as cobalamin because it contains cobalt. It is a member of the water-soluble B complex family and is sometimes known as 'anti-pernicious' factor because it prevents pernicious anaemia.

Vitamin B12 is needed at a very basic level for the synthesis of DNA and hence for cell production – particularly red blood cells (see also iron).

This vitamin is lost in cooking water and also sensitive to strong acid, alkali and light, so if your diet is too acidic (for example if you eat a lot of meat and/or bread and not enough vegetables), vitamin B12 will not be available to your body.

Signs of B12 deficiency are (Mervyn 1989):

- pernicious anaemia

- smooth, sore tongue

- moodiness

- poor memory

- paranoia

- mental confusion

- tiredness

- menstrual disorders

- poor appetite.

Vitamin B12 deficiency can be brought on by parasites (see Chapter 5), vegetarianism, old age, pregnancy, alcohol and smoking.

This vitamin is only available through animal protein, although there is some in spirulina.

Vitamin B12 is water-soluble and can be taken with or without food.

Folic acid

Folic acid is one of the B vitamins and, just like vitamin B12 and iron, helps prevent and reverse anaemia. It is needed for blood formation, genetic code transmission and resistance to infections.

If you are deficient in folic acid, you can develop any of the following symptoms:

- anaemia

- decrease in white blood cells (lowered immune responses)

- weakness

- fatigue

- breathlessness

- irritability

- insomnia

- mental confusion

- forgetfulness.

Folic acid robbers are alcohol, pregnancy, the contraceptive pill and many pharmaceutical drugs as well as drugs used in the treatment of cancer.

If you are on anti-epileptic drugs, you should not take folic acid without consulting your doctor first. Folic acid can mask a deficiency of vitamin B12, so it is important to check whether your B12 levels are sufficient before starting to take folic acid.

Folic acid is a member of the B vitamin family and is water-soluble. You can take it with or without food.

Further information

BOOKS

Brewer, S. (2002) *The Daily Telegraph Encyclopaedia of Vitamins, Minerals and Herbal Supplements*. London: Daily Telegraph.

A very good A–Z review of vitamins, minerals and herbal supplements which explains the benefits, possible side-effects and contraindications. It also cites research and has a separate section where you can look up illnesses and which supplements are recommended.

USEFUL ADDRESSES

HGUK hair sample testing (see p.20)

Remedy #8: Detox body and scalp

When hair starts falling out suddenly or when hair is shed in much larger quantities than normal, you need to look at what is interfering with your general health. As all the body processes are closely interlinked, it is often not enough just to use a topical product on the scalp, as the real problem is happening within the entire body system.

In a previous chapter, you read about the dangers of amalgam fillings and heavy metals in the body and how they can lead to hormonal imbalance and persistent parasite infestation. The obvious solution is to have the source of toxicity removed, but that in itself is not enough. You will also have to help the body get rid of the metals from the tissues and clean the whole digestive tract of the parasites which have had a free-for-all up until now!

There are a great many natural remedies that can help you achieve this detoxification, but not all of them will suit you or be right for you. It is also important that you take the right quantity of an indicated supplement and that you take it for long enough really to get the body cleansed of the toxins it is holding.

Detoxifying the liver

We all build up toxins in the liver over the years, and this stops the body from functioning as well as it could. Fillings in your teeth, vaccinations, medical or recreational drugs, too much fat and sugar in the diet as well as pollutants in the air and the water all contribute to the toxic load on liver and kidneys.

The following symptoms may be an indication that your liver is not working as it should (www.britishlivertrust.org.uk; www.merckmanuals.com):

- right shoulder stiffness, tightness or soreness
- feeling irritable/stressed a lot of the time
- fuzzy or foggy vision
- headaches
- poor concentration
- itchy, irritated, red or dry eyes
- insomnia, restless or interrupted sleep
- irritability and impatience
- hot flushes
- dry, bad, itchy, burning or irritated skin
- a constant itch that never goes away
- muddled thinking
- overwhelming moods or emotions
- wound up and ready to explode
- liver issues
- gallbladder flare-ups
- craving alcohol
- nose, sinus or chest congestion
- acne, boils, rashes or breakouts.

All these can be symptoms of a clogged-up liver. Even if you have only three of the above symptoms, you should do a liver cleanse.

The following liver cleanse will help you get rid of the toxin build up in the liver and kidneys. It is also very effective in breaking down cholesterol in the bloodstream by preventing fatty deposits from forming along the walls of the arteries. Virgin olive oil is a mono-unsaturated fat which does not clog the arteries or contain cholesterol. It also increases the body's levels of high density lipoproteins (HDL) or 'good cholesterol'. The HDL allows the blood to absorb more cholesterol so that it can be eliminated by the liver.

LIVER CLEANSE
You will need:

- 100 ml freshly squeezed lemon juice (approx. two ripe lemons)

- 100 ml bottled or filtered still water

- organic apple juice

- 1 tablespoon extra-virgin olive oil

- garlic supplement from the health food shop (any brand)

- peppermint tea.

1. Mix the lemon juice, water and olive oil together and add a dash of apple juice. Drink this mixture first thing in the morning on an empty stomach. With the drink, take a garlic capsule.

   If you find it difficult to consume the above amount of lemon juice, top up your drink with more organic apple juice or use a straw to drink the mixture.

2. Fifteen minutes after having drunk the liver cleanse drink, have a hot cup of peppermint tea. *Drink plenty of water* throughout the day – at least eight large glasses – and eat light meals only on the day of the liver cleanse, avoiding fatty foods such as milk products and red meats.

3. Repeat this detox three days in a row.

Detoxing for metals

Caution: If you are pregnant, breastfeeding or planning a pregnancy, or if you are on prescribed medication, do not take any of the following supplements unless prescribed by a qualified health practitioner.

CHLORELLA

Chlorella is a sea-moss which contains high levels of chlorophyll and more vitamin B12 than liver (Bartram 1998). It produces protein 50 times more efficiently than other crops, including soya and rice. It contains 19 of the 22 amino acids, including the eight essentials. It is a rich source of DNA/RNA and of calcium, iron, selenium and zinc. It is a potent liver detoxifier, and it is antibiotic and a metabolic stimulant. It cleanses the bowels while at the same time providing nutrients for friendly gut flora. It is anti-viral, anti-candida and a fat mobiliser. It has been shown to have a high binding affinity for poisonous substances in the gut and liver.

Please note: not everyone tolerates chlorella, so if you take it, only take a small amount to prevent a severe detox reaction.

CHARCOAL

Charcoal has not only the power to neutralise putrid smells of cancer, diarrhoea and gangrene, but it also has a great capacity for absorbing gases and bacterial toxins. Taking one or several charcoal tablets on the day that you are having amalgam fillings replaced is a good way of ensuring that the toxic fumes released during dental treatment are absorbed and carried out of the body (McTaggart 2006). You may have to continue with charcoal for a few days afterwards.

ZINC

Zinc is an important element in the healthy absorption and function of vitamins, especially the B-complex vitamins (Leonard 1989; Peraza *et al.* 1998). It is involved in digestion and metabolism, as well as contributing to tissue growth, maintenance and repair. Zinc is destroyed when food is processed, and low levels of zinc are common today. Zinc deficiencies can lead to abnormalities of sense and perception (loss of smell or taste), increased risk of infection, lethargy, malfunctioning sex glands and poor appetite. Zinc is vital to a healthy immune system because it speeds the healing of wounds and assists thymus function. If you eat lots of fibre, this will deplete your zinc levels. You should also supplement zinc if you are vegetarian or eat little meat, or if you are on a calorie-reduced diet.

Please note. If you still have amalgam fillings in your teeth, only take zinc in small amounts (15 mg per day maximum) to avoid the mercury becoming 'cemented' into the body.

SELENIUM

Selenium is an important mineral which works together with vitamin E to carry out many metabolic functions, including normal growth and fertility (Lindh, Danersund and Lindvall 1996; Psarras, Derand and Nilner 1994). It is a powerful antioxidant and anti-cancer nutrient. It is known to guard the body from numerous disorders, including arteriosclerosis, coronary artery disease, heart attacks and strokes. Selenium can be found in many vegetables such as broccoli, cauliflower, garlic, onions and radishes. However, the selenium content in food is dependent on the amount of selenium in the soils where the food is grown, so chances are you need to supplement it as our soils today are generally of poor quality.

VITAMIN C

Vitamin C, also known as ascorbic acid, is a water-soluble substance which must be obtained from dietary sources. Vitamin C helps form red blood cells, aids in the prevention of haemorrhaging and enhances fine bone and tooth formation. It is also necessary for the functioning of other essential nutrients in the body. Intestinal absorption of iron is significantly increased by sufficient levels of vitamin C. It has been clinically proven to decrease the intensity of colds substantially and to help in preventing cancer (Mamede *et al.* 2012). An adequate amount of vitamin C is vital for the creation of adrenalin in the adrenal glands. Adrenal ascorbic acid is quickly used up in times of stress and it is therefore important to replenish it regularly. Take vitamin C in divided doses throughout the day to ensure consistent levels in the blood as vitamin C is quickly excreted from the body. Take between 1000 and 3000 mg when you are stressed. If you get diarrhoea it means that you have exceeded your optimum level. Simply reduce your intake by 500 mg.

VITAMIN E

Vitamin E is indispensable to all oxygen-breathing life and is an intricate component of energy production. Vitamin E is fat-soluble and is made up of several substances called tocopherols. It is a powerful anti-oxidant which plays a vital role in the cellular respiration of all muscles, particularly cardiac and skeletal. It enables these muscles and associated nerves to operate with less oxygen, thus enhancing their endurance and stamina. Sufficient levels of vitamin E are essential for healthy neurological functioning – a deficiency can often cause nerve damage. Vitamin E improves blood flow by dilating blood vessels, inhibits blood clotting, transports nutrients to cells, assists eye focus, promotes healing of wounds and reduces scarring, and protects the body against damage from environmental pollutants. It can be derived from food sources such as whole-grain cereals, all raw seeds and nuts, eggs, vegetables (especially leafy greens) and cold-pressed vegetable oils. Take together with selenium. As this vitamin is fat-soluble, it is best taken with food.

Please note: Vitamin E is often made with soy. If you suspect you are intolerant to soy, choose a supplement that is made without soy.

L-CYSTEINE

Cysteine is a water-soluble sulphur amino acid that is a biochemical powerhouse. Its most exciting trait is its ability to help the body rid itself of harmful toxic chemicals such as mercury, as well as toxins which occur in cancer treatments. In itself, cysteine is also used in combating cancer. Apart from helping with metal toxicity, cysteine also plays a role in energy metabolism and has been successfully used in the treatment of hair loss in women, in psoriasis and in cases of bacterial infection (Braverman *et al.* 1997).

L-cysteine is an amino acid and has to be taken at least half an hour away from food, ideally on an empty stomach.

L-GLUTATHIONE

There are virtually no living organisms – animal or plant – whose cells don't contain some glutathione. Scientists believe that glutathione was essential to the very development of life on earth (Braverman *et al.* 1997). Liver, spleen, kidneys, stomach lining, pancreas and the eyes contain the greatest amount of glutathione. The amount of glutathione in the body decreases with age.

Glutathione plays four primary roles in the body. It protects against powerful man-made oxidants, it helps the liver detoxify poisonous chemicals, it supports immune function and protects the integrity of red blood cells. It is able to bind and remove metals such as lead, mercury, arsenic and cadmium.

L-glutathione is an amino acid and has to be taken at least half an hour away from food, ideally on an empty stomach.

N-ACETYL-L CYSTEINE (NAC)

NAC is able to antidote more toxins than any other substance in the body. NAC is used in emergency rooms against toxic overdose and has been used successfully to deal with pulmonary problems, cancer and heart conditions. The immune system is particularly sensitive to a deficiency of NAC, so if you suffer from an auto-immune disorder, you may need to supplement with NAC. NAC also improves eradication of heliobacter pylori bacteria and is documented as being a powerful antidote for arsenic and mercury poisoning (Braverman *et al.* 1997).

NAC is an amino acid and has to be taken at least half an hour away from food, ideally on an empty stomach.

SARSAPARILLA

Sarsaparilla is a herb which has anti-inflammatory, antiseptic and anti-rheumatic properties. It is a metabolic stimulant and an immune enhancer. It is a pituitary stimulant and substitute for adrenal steroid. It has been used successfully in cases of mercury poisoning, bacterial dysentery, psoriasis, eczema and PMT.

Detoxing for parasites

Caution: If you are pregnant, breastfeeding or planning a pregnancy, or if you are on prescribed medication, do not take any of the following herbs unless prescribed by a qualified health practitioner.

GOLDENSEAL

Goldenseal increases the secretion of digestive enzymes and fluids, especially bile, which helps regulate liver and spleen functions. The berberine contained in goldenseal has been studied at length for its antibacterial and amoebicidal properties (Wu *et al.* 2012; Yan *et al.* 2012). If you suffer from hypoglycaemia, use goldenseal only under the supervision of a health practitioner as it may lower blood sugar levels.

OREGON GRAPE

Oregon grape is a close relative of barberry. It enhances glandular function, especially of the liver and the thyroid, improves digestion and absorption of nutrients, purifies the blood and even shrinks certain tumours. Like goldenseal, oregon grape is a good source of berberine. It helps enhance the production of bile which assists the liver in eliminating toxins. It has antibiotic effects, as well as being antibacterial.

BARBERRY

Barberry bark is a liver stimulant. It is antiseptic and a tonic to the spleen and pancreas. It helps fight inflammation and has a history of being effective against bacteria and amoebae.

GARLIC

Garlic is another plant with antibiotic qualities. It is helpful in eliminating parasites of any description and also has anti-tumour properties. It contains B vitamins (which are vital for hair growth) as well as minerals. It has also a good track record in the fight against candidiasis and other fungal infections.

BLACK WALNUT

Black walnut has been used to expel a variety of intestinal parasites, worms and yeast. External applications of black walnut have been shown to kill ringworm, while Chinese herbalists use this herb to eliminate tapeworms from the body. It also helps heal eczema and psoriasis.

WORMWOOD

Wormwood is a potent anti-parasitic which also helps fight inflammation. It is particularly useful if your liver is not working efficiently as it helps stimulate bile and promotes stomach acid production. Wormwood should only be taken or used with cold water, as hot water will wipe out its beneficial effects.

CLOVES

Cloves are a spice which, taken as a supplement, has powerful antiseptic qualities. The remedy is used for flatulence, diarrhoea, worms and externally as essential oil for asthma, bronchitis, pleurisy and lung conditions.

PAU D'ARCO

Pau d'Arco is a powerful anti-fungal and has the reputation of curing certain forms of candidiasis, ringworm and other intestinal parasite infestations. It has also been successfully used in the treatment of cancer without causing any of the adverse effects generated by conventional cancer treatment.

Further information

BOOKS

Bartram, T. (1998) *Bartram's Encyclopaedia of Herbal Medicine.* London: Robinson.

An excellent book which gives the therapeutic properties of herbs, and also lists various illnesses and which herbs can help. Highly recommended.

Braverman, E.R. (1997) *The Healing Nutrients Within.* Canaan, CT: Keats Publishing.

All about essential and non-essential amino acids and their clinical uses in counteracting illnesses.

USEFUL ADDRESSES

Health Kinesiology UK
www.hk4health.co.uk
+44 (0)8707 655 980

HGUK hair sample testing to find out exactly what you need to take (see p.20)

Remedy #9: Exercises that help hair growth

I have noticed with many of my clients that they are quite stiff around the shoulder and neck region. This is a problem, not just because of the pain and discomfort it can cause, but also because it can adversely influence hair growth.

In order for hair follicles to be nourished adequately, there has to be good circulation in the scalp area. It is the circulation of blood that brings the necessary nutrients to the hair follicles to help them grow.

This, however, can only happen if neck and shoulders are loose and comfortable.

You may already be aware of the need for good scalp circulation and may therefore massage your scalp regularly, and this is a good thing to do. However, this will not have a beneficial effect unless neck and shoulders are relaxed as well. With tight neck and shoulders, all you are doing by massaging the scalp is to shuffle the stagnant blood in the scalp around a bit, but not enough oxygenated blood is coming through to the scalp to make a difference because the neck and shoulders are 'blocked'.

Another reason why a tight neck and shoulder region is a problem for hair growth is that cellular debris and toxins are getting stuck in the scalp area rather than being moved on. These toxins can then prevent the hair follicles from developing normally.

A tight neck or tense shoulders will automatically mean tight scalp muscles. Anything that is tight suppresses proper blood supply.

The following exercises are crucial if any of the following points apply to you:

- you have just lived through a very stressful period of your life

- you are often stressed

- you are of a nervous disposition or suffer with anxiety

- you have a sedentary job

- you have had a lot of dental work done in your life

- you don't do any exercise

- you exercise mainly your legs and lower body.

Check whether your neck and shoulders are stiff.

A simple way of checking whether you have a problem with shoulders and/or neck is to try the following:

Test l

- Put your right hand on your left shoulder, just where your neck begins, and gently push your fingers into the top of your left shoulder.

- Gently increase the pressure until your fingers are dug into the shoulder.

- Now move your fingers from the top of your left shoulder down to where your left arm starts.

- Repeat the test with your left hand on your right shoulder.

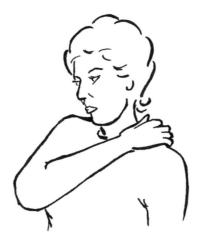

Figure 3 Testing for stiffness in neck and shoulders

Does any of this hurt? – If it does, you have a problem.

Some people have a problem with only one shoulder. In my experience, a problem with the left shoulder signifies that you are not breathing properly, whereas pain in the right shoulder can mean that you have a problem with your liver.

Test 2

- Stand up straight and push your shoulders down as much as you can.

Does this hurt? – If it does, you have a problem.

Test 3

- Stand or sit up straight.

- Slowly and gently begin to turn your head to the right, as if you were trying to look over your right shoulder. Make sure you only move your head, not the rest of your body.

Does the left or right side of your neck hurt? – If it does, you have a problem.

- Repeat the test now, turning your head to the left, as if you were trying to look over your left shoulder without moving the rest of your body.

Does the left or right side of your neck hurt? – If it does, you have a problem.

You may find that only one side of your neck hurts, no matter whether you turn your neck to the left or to the right. This may be an indication that you have a faulty bite on that side of the mouth.

How a faulty bite can affect the rest of your body

If you are having problems with your neck or your shoulders, this can indicate that your upper jaw does not fit properly onto your lower jaw. This can be caused if the temporo-mandibular joint (TMJ) is out of alignment.

The TMJ is the joint that connects your lower jaw and your skull. The movement in the TMJ allows you to open and close your mouth and to chew from side to side. To find your TMJ, touch the area of your face just in front of your ears and open and close your mouth. The TMJ is the area that moves up and down when your lower jaw opens and closes.

One reason why the TMJ can be out of alignment is if you have had a lot of dental work done where you had to keep your mouth wide open for a long time. Another reason can be that you have had orthodontic treatment which helped line up your teeth nicely but left your TMJ in the wrong position.

A faulty bite can cause any of the following problems (private interview with Dr Ljuba Lemke DMD, 2005; see www. holistichealthsource.com):

- teeth are out of line, heavily worn or constantly breaking

- fillings fracture or crowns work loose

- teeth hurt when biting food or ache constantly, even without eating

- teeth become loose
- receding gums get worse
- clicking or pain in the jaw joints
- grinding teeth at night or when concentrating
- ringing or buzzing in the ears
- difficulty in opening or closing your mouth
- muscle spasms in your jaws
- headaches or migraines, especially first thing in the morning
- pain behind the eyes, sinus pain
- pain in neck and shoulders
- back muscles ache.

The exercises

Even if you only do one of the following exercises, you will help your neck and shoulders relax more. Relaxed neck and shoulders help scalp muscles relax, and this in turn will help increase the blood supply to the scalp.

Some general rules apply to the following exercises.

- Do the exercises in the order described here. That way, you get a warm up first before you start using body strength.

- If you only do one exercise, do the first one.

- Start with a number of repeats that are comfortable, then gradually increase the repeats as you become stronger and more used to the exercises.

Exercise 1: Backward circles

1. Drink a glass of water.

2. Stand on a mini-trampoline or on your bed.

3. Gently start bouncing, but don't let your feet leave the surface of the trampoline or bed.

4. Hold your arms out to your sides at shoulder height and start making small circles backwards with your hands. Do as many circles backwards as you can manage comfortably, then do five more.

5. You should aim for about 100 rotations, but start with as few as you want to and build up slowly.

6. When you have finished, drink another glass of water.

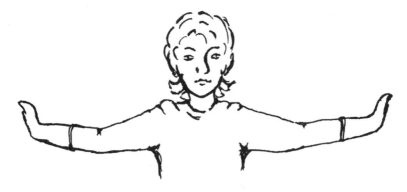

Figure 4 Backward circles exercise

DURATION
Approximately 1 minute.

AIM
To loosen the shoulders and increase circulation from the trunk of the body into the neck and scalp.

Bouncing will get your lymph moving so that toxins can be carried out of the body with the aid of the water you have just drunk.

TIPS
- If you can't feel your shoulder blades move, push your outstretched arms a bit further back behind you when you make circles with your hands.

- If you hold your arms out with your fingertips pointing upwards you will increase the effect of the exercise.

Exercise 2: Easy push-ups

I can already hear you groaning, but don't worry – even I can do this exercise, and I've never been to a gym in my life!

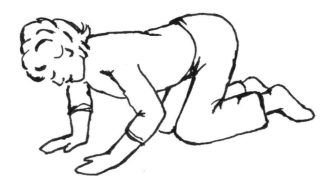

Figure 5 Easy push-ups exercise

1. Kneel on the floor, hands in front of you, as if you were a table.

2. Lower your upper body halfway towards the floor and come up again.

3. Do as many push-ups as you can, then do one more.

4. Aim eventually to do 50, but build up slowly from day to day.

DURATION
Approximately 1 minute.

AIM
To increase circulation in the shoulders and push more blood into the neck and scalp regions.

TIP

- Do the Easy Push-ups immediately after the Backward Circles. You will notice that you can do more push-ups when your shoulders are warmed up by the arm rolls.

Exercise 3: Stretch up

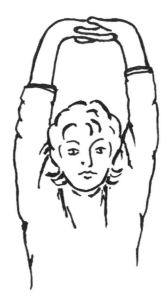

Figure 6 Stretch-up exercise

1. Stand up straight and fold your hands.

2. Keep your fingers interlinked and turn your folded hands so that your palms point outwards.

3. Stretch out your arms above your head, fingers still interlinked and palms facing the ceiling.

4. Hold this stretch with arms as straight as possible for a count of 60 or as long as you can.

5. Don't forget to breathe!

6. Eventually, aim to hold your arms up in a Stretch Up position for the count of 120.

DURATION

Approximately 1–2 minutes.

AIM

To make arm muscles more supple, raise up the shoulder blades and increase circulation to the neck and scalp.

TIP

- If you cannot stretch out your arms all the way, leave them a little bent. That's OK. After practising for a while, you'll get more supple.

Exercise 4: Relaxing the TMJ

The following exercise is very important to do if you suffer from any of the TMJ-related complaints listed earlier.

To start off with, locate your temporo-mandibular joint (TMJ) again by touching the area of your face just in front of your ears and open and close your mouth slightly.

1. Drink a glass of water before starting this exercise.

2. Sit comfortably, ideally in a way where both your back and head are supported.

3. Cup your face in your hands, with the palms of your hands covering your lower jaws and your fingers covering your ears.

4. With upper and lower teeth slightly apart, lips slightly open, keep your face cupped as described in step 3 and stay like this to the count of 60.

5. Now let your mouth drop open wide while still holding your face cupped as before. Hold this position to the count of 60.

6. Over time, increase steps 4 and 5 to the count of 120 each.

7. Drink another glass of water.

DURATION

Between 2 and 4 minutes.

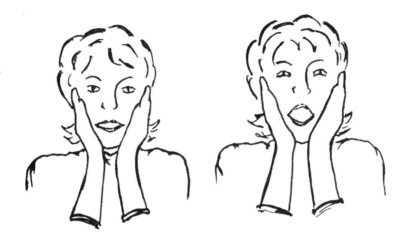

Figure 7 Relaxing the TMJ exercise

AIM

To allow the TMJ to re-align itself again.

This exercise also has a detoxifying effect on the facial area. As you are allowing the jaw muscles to relax, the toxins trapped in the facial and scalp tissue can start being released.

TIP

- You can increase the effectiveness of this exercise if you imagine that your left and your right TMJ are linked by an elastic thread that goes horizontally through your mouth.

Further information

Philip Rafferty RESET

www.kinergetics.com.au

www.reset-tmj.com

Philip Rafferty has a system of relaxing jaw muscles with some simple exercises which enables the TMJ to reset. The methods can be learnt in a three-hour workshop. His excellent little book *RESET 1* is possibly no longer in print, but if you can get hold of it, I recommend it.

Remedy #10: Stimulate and cleanse hair follicles

If your hair has only started falling out recently or if it has started regrowing but does so only very slowly, you can help it along by stimulating the scalp. There are various ways in which you can do that.

Hair and scalp care

Wash your head regularly every two or three days, even if you have no hair. It is important that you keep the hair follicles unclogged so that your hair has no obstacles in its way once it starts growing again.

Use jojoba oil to keep the pores and hair follicles free of dead skin cells. Apply a quarter of a teaspoon of the oil to your scalp and gently massage it into the skin without pulling the skin or pressing hard into the scalp. You can do this in the evening and leave it on overnight. If you have no hair, you can put a cotton turban on your head at night or put a towel over your pillow if you are worried that the oil will stain your bedclothes. In my experience, this doesn't happen though.

To wash your hair or scalp, buy loose nettle tea. Take a handful and boil it in water. Strain the tea through a sieve and use the cooled down nettle water to wash your hair in. Nettles stimulate hair growth.

Alternatively, use a shampoo, but avoid the following ingredients as they are a *health hazard*:

SODIUM LAURYL SULPHATE (SLS) AND SODIUM LAURETH SULPHATE (SLES)

These are industrial degreasers and can cause flaky skin and hair loss.

DIETHANOLAMINE (DEA)

This substance is a potential carcinogen, even in small doses. Repeated use of DEA increases the risk of cancer (Andrew *et al.* 2004; McTaggart 2003).

PROPYLENE GLYCOL (PG) OR ISOPROPYL ALCOHOL

PG can lead to rashes, dry skin and dermatitis. Not what you need if your hair is already having problems growing properly! Isopropyl alcohol is associated with cancer, so avoid it. (Dhillon and von Burg 1995)

PARABENS

Methyl, propyl, butyl and ethyl parabens are toxic and can cause rashes and other allergic reactions.

Don't be fooled by the word 'natural' on hair products – that does not mean they don't have the above substances in them. Start reading labels!

Hair dyes

By the way, while you are having problems with your hair, be very careful which hair dyes you use. The majority of dyes are toxic and can aggravate hair loss. Especially black, dark-brown and red shade hair dyes are associated with cancer (Shafer and Shafer 1976; Shore *et al.* 1979).

In hair dyes, the following ingredients are a health hazard:

- octynoic acid

- toluidine

- p-aminophenol.

These three ingredients are suspected of causing liver damage.

PARA-PHENYLENEDIAMINE (PPD)

This ingredient is a colourant which penetrates the hair shaft and follicle, and it also has a strong protein-binding capacity. This makes PPD an ideal contact allergen. Allergic reactions to PPD have become such a serious problem that the chemical has been banned completely from hair dyes in Germany, France and Sweden.

Once you have a contact allergy triggered by PPD, you can develop a rash on your face or around the hairline, swelling of the face, scalp and ears.

PPD accumulates in skin over time and can lead to cross-sensitisation which means that you can become sensitive to other chemicals as well.

PPD is also contained in black 'henna' skin paint for temporary tattoos.

RESORCIN

This substance is absorbed through the skin into the body and can trigger allergies. There are also indications that it causes liver and kidney damage.

POLYETHYLENE GLYCOL/PEG

PEG compounds have been found to contain ethylene oxide which is linked to breast and other cancers. They have also been found to contain heavy metals such as arsenic (which causes hair loss), lead (which causes hair loss), iron, cadmium and cobalt.

So my message is: Read labels, read labels, read labels!

Further information

GOOD MAKES FOR HAIR AND BODY PRODUCTS ARE:

Aubrey Organics
www.aubreyorganicsuk.co.uk
www.aubrey-organics.com
Australia: from www.innerglow.com.au
+44 (0)20 8688 2366

Avalon Organics
www.avalonorganics.com
USA: www.iHerb.com
Australia: www.organicsaustraliaonline.com.au
New Zealand: www.mynaturalhealth.co.nz
+1 888 659 7730

Barefoot Botanicals
www.barefootbotanicals.com
+44 (0)1273 325666

Faith in Nature
www.faithinnature.co.uk
+44 (0)161 724 4016

Handmade Naturals
www.handmadenaturals.co.uk
+44 (0)1270 877 516

SAFE HAIR DYES

Aubrey Organics Colour Me Natural
www.aubreyorganicsuk.co.uk
www.aubrey-organics.com
Australia: from www.innerglow.com.au
+44 (0)20 8688 2366

Logona Natural Hair Dyes
Available from Suvarna
+44 (0)1695 728286

Stimulate the scalp

This is a good thing to do, and it's quite OK to press very firmly as you massage.

Massage with your head hanging down, and massage from the back of your neck up to the crown, then from the sides of your head up to the top, then from the hairline at the front up to the top of your head.

The good thing about massaging the scalp is that it not only gets the circulation to your scalp going, but it also makes you raise your arms, and that helps the shoulders get a little workout too so that the circulation is increased in the upper body as well.

Another way of stimulating the scalp is with herbal gels or oils. If you buy anything over the counter, it is likely to cost a lot and be full of chemicals that will not simply stay on your scalp but wander into your body. It is simpler to make up your own recipe which is cheap and natural. There are a number of oils and gels that are very good for the scalp and hair growth.

- *Aloe vera gel* is antiviral, antibacterial and a precursor of vitamin B12. It is particularly effective if you have just started developing alopecia areata bald patches or if you have hair loss due to ringworm. Use twice a day.

- *Olive oil* stimulates strong hair growth. Gently massage a couple of drops into the scalp. Use twice a day.

- *Jojoba oil* helps keep the follicles clean which is very important. Put one or two drops of rosemary essential oil into three tablespoons of jojoba to give it a stimulating effect. Keep the oil in a cool, dark place. Apply a few drops of this mixture to your scalp and leave on overnight. Use twice a week.

  Only use a few drops of the essential oil, and NEVER use it undiluted.

- *Apple cider vinegar* helps normalise the pH balance of the skin and keeps bacteria at bay. Leave on head for 15 minutes or overnight, then shampoo hair/head. If the smell is too strong, dilute the vinegar with water. Use once a day.

Now comes the really important bit – get yourself a metal comb or a hairbrush with metal teeth and gently tap all over your head with it. Do this for about a minute, ideally after you have done your scalp relaxing exercises (see earlier in this chapter) so that overall circulation is good and your shoulders and neck are loose.

The reason why it is very important that you use a comb or brush with metal teeth is that the tapping with metal will create tiny electromagnetic currents on the scalp which stimulate the cells in the hair follicles. Tapping with a horn or plastic comb will stimulate the circulation but won't create the electromagnetic currents.

HAIR BRUSHING

You may remember the age-old advice to brush your hair 100 times every day. If your hair is healthy, the brushing motion with any brush, even if it is not metal, will generate a lot of electricity, and this stimulates the hair follicles.

To get the maximum effect from hair brushing, you can use a magnetic hairbrush which heightens the beneficial effect on the scalp and hair follicles.

There is also a machine available that fulfils a similar function. It is called an electrotrichogenesis machine (ETG) and is used by some trichologists as a way of making hair grow faster once it has started regrowing again.

ETG employs electrical stimulation to promote cellular activity in the hair follicles with a pulsed electrical field. The patient sits under a device that resembles a beauty salon hairdryer. Inside the hood are four pairs of positively and negatively charged electrodes, powered by a 12-volt battery, positioned between 1 and 5 centimetres from the person's head. When the machine is turned on, the person's scalp is bathed in an electric field for about 10–12 minutes. In order to receive this treatment, you need to see a trichologist or dermatologist who has access to an ETG machine.

An article in the *International Journal of Dermatology* reported reasonably good results for men, although treatment only worked for people who have had hair problems for a relatively short time. Treatment has to be kept up for life to keep up the benefits, so it's not something that I would recommend unless you have found the underlying cause for the hair loss and have rectified it and your hair has started growing again. If this is the case, the ETG treatment can speed up the rate of hair growth considerably.

You will also see laser treatment advertised which claims to help hair regrow. Again, you are put under a type of hairdryer contraption, only this time the machine emits laser beams. This is new and no long-term studies exist. Please be careful – we do not know about potential side-effects on the brain.

Further information

MAGNETIC HAIRBRUSH FROM

Magnetic Therapy Ltd
www.magnetictherapy.co.uk
+44 (0)845 130 5110
This company delivers to Europe, America, Canada and Australia.

ETG TREATMENT

To find out whether ETG treatment is available in your area, you will need to go and speak to a trichologist or contact:

The Institute of Trichologists
www.trichologists.org.uk
+44 (0)1302 380028

National Trichology Training Institute
www.nttiga.com

CHAPTER 7

HOW THERAPIES CAN HELP

You may feel that your hair loss problem has been going on for too long, and you are not too confident about tackling it with the self-help methods that I outlined in the previous chapters. This is fine. Not everyone is a 'DIY' fan!

In order to help you find someone who can check conditions such as metal poisoning and parasites for you and sort out any other underlying causes of your hair loss, I have put together information about a number of therapies that can help.

I'm sure that the following list of natural therapies is not comprehensive. There will be many more types of natural therapies that have successfully treated clients with hair loss problems. The fact that only a few are mentioned here is simply a reflection of my limited knowledge and is in no way meant to be disrespectful or dismissive of any other therapies.

If you are a therapist reading this book whose branch of natural therapy is not mentioned in the following pages, and if you have had good results with more than two clients with serious hair loss problems, please write to me so that I can include your type of therapy in future publications. Contact details are at the back of the book.

Treatment #1: Hair or nail sample tests

You will have read throughout the book references to HGUK hair or nail sample tests which can help discover whether you have toxins in your body or not. These tests can also tell you exactly which supplements you need to take in order to detox, to support hair growth or to generally bring the body back to health.

I would like to explain a little more about the HGUK tests as they are different from conventional laboratory tests.

Each part of the body, each organ and each gland, each living and dead thing has its own unique frequency pattern. Every single cell in the body contains your DNA, and each cell of the body, including your hair, reflects the total energy frequency of the whole person. As hair is the easiest set of cells to remove from the body, it is one of the most convenient ways of obtaining a sample for analysis.

If the vitamin or mineral content in your body needs to be determined, a laboratory is able to analyse your hair sample and give you precise feedback on the amounts of, for example, zinc in your body. If you are deficient and the lab works together with a nutritionist, they will give you a general recommendation regarding how much zinc you should take to top up your reserves. If they don't work with a nutritionist, they'll only tell you that you are deficient and it is up to you to do something about it.

With HGUK testing, you won't get a precise figure of your zinc body content. Testing can only tell you whether your body is short of zinc or not. What it *can* determine much more precisely than a laboratory or nutritionist is exactly how much you have to take, how often a day and for how many weeks you have to take the zinc to make up for that deficiency. The difference between laboratory testing and HGUK testing is that the laboratory is more exact concerning the deficiency status quo whereas HGUK testing is more precise about how to remedy the deficiency.

Another difference between laboratory and kinesiology testing is that laboratories can often not find parasites as these are notoriously hard to detect. The lab might get a stool sample from you which does not contain any evidence of parasites even though you have parasites in your body. Also, certain parasites cannot be detected with traditional laboratory tests at all.

HGUK testing can test for all parasites, provided the relevant test vial is in my test kit. I am not looking for the physical presence of a parasite in your hair sample but for the unique energy frequencies of that parasite. So even if the parasite hides in the bloodstream or in an organ, their vibrational pattern can still be detected in a hair sample.

There is a similar issue with toxic metals where conventional laboratory testing is concerned. Checking the urine or blood will not always reveal whether you have, for example, mercury in your system. Depending on your state of health at the time of testing, toxic metals do not show up in your blood or urine sample. Metals are often deposited in organs and adipose (fatty) tissues in the body because the body does not know what to do with them. This means a laboratory test cannot detect them in your blood or urine.

If you are not very stressed, the toxic metal stays in the tissues. Only when you get stressed or exert yourself physically, the toxins get released back into the bloodstream where they can be detected by conventional laboratory testing. So getting an 'all clear' from a laboratory does not mean that you have no toxic metals. It means that they were not able to find any. Testing a hair sample with HGUK kinesiology methods however will reveal the metals because the frequency of the metal can be detected, no matter where in the body the metal is located.

Taking a hair sample is easy. Simply cut off about ten hairs from the nape of your neck, as near to the scalp as possible. It does not matter if your hair is dyed. The hairs should be about 2 centimetres long or longer. You *must not* take hair from a brush or comb as this might contain someone else's hair and consequently confuse the issue.

If you have no hair or your hair is too short, you can instead take clippings from your fingernails (without nail varnish on them). The larger you can make the clippings, the better. If in doubt, take little clippings from several nails.

Put your sample into a piece of paper, fold the paper over a few times and write your name on the paper.

There is also an extensive questionnaire where, among many other things, you will be asked for the following information:

- Are you currently taking any medications? (The supplements could interfere with your medication.)

- Are you pregnant, breastfeeding or planning on becoming pregnant? (If you are, I can only check for toxicities but will not test any supplements for you until a time when you have weaned your baby.)

Further information
HGUK tests (see p.20)

Vera PeifferHairgrowthUK™®

Treatment #2: Health kinesiology

Health kinesiology (HK) has been around for over 20 years. It was devised by Dr Jimmy Scott, a physiological psychologist who initially specialised in biofeedback research at the University of California Medical School.

HK is a combination of traditional Chinese medicine and Western style muscle testing. An HK practitioner uses acupuncture points on their client's body to establish where the client's energy system is weak. By touching an acupuncture point on the client's body and at the same time exerting gentle pressure on, say, the client's arm muscle, a biofeedback is established. If the arm muscle weakens, it tells the practitioner that there is a problem relating to that particular acupuncture point. If the arm muscle stays strong, the practitioner knows that the energy is flowing freely through that particular acupuncture point. They can then move on to test various other points in the same way.

Each acupuncture point is related to a particular meridian. Meridians are energy pathways that flow through the body, just below the surface of the skin, with every meridian serving a particular organ or gland. If the energy cannot flow freely through the meridian, the related organ or gland will not get the energy it needs to be fully functional. In the long run, this can lead to ill health or disease.

HK can help with a great number of psychological and physical problems. It is an ideal tool to discover whether you have an allergy or intolerance to certain foods, additives, common metals or other substances. It can also test whether you have bacteria, fungi, parasites or moulds in your body as well as finding out which remedies or supplements are necessary to get rid of them.

In order to establish whether you have an intolerance, a small glass vial containing that substance is placed on your body while the HK practitioner gently presses on your arm. If your arm goes down, you have an intolerance to that substance. The weakened arm muscle is a sign that your body gets stressed when it has the substance anywhere near it, and this is a sign of intolerance or allergy.

But HK can go even further. A number of procedures can actually help heighten your tolerance level to an allergen so that you are able to tolerate the substance again after a while.

HK stimulates energy flow and encourages detoxification, and as the body gets rid of accumulated waste, nutrients can get to the cells and help heal the body.

In the context of hair loss, HK can help discover what is at the bottom of your problem. When you first speak to an HK practitioner on the phone, make sure that they have the following test kits:

- foods A, B and C

- invasive organisms

- common metals.

I have personally trained kinesiologists to deal with hair loss problems who have these test kits. To find a list of these practitioners, please go to my website.

In addition to testing for and correcting allergies and intolerances, HK can also help the body absorb nutrients better. In some cases, I have observed that clients were unable to absorb certain minerals. Even though these clients were taking all the right supplements, their cells were unable to utilise them. This, however, can be remedied with a variety of procedures (see also Jane Thurnell-Read's book on health kinesiology).

What happens in an HK session?

You will be asked to lie on a couch fully clothed but without your shoes. The HK practitioner will then use a muscle on your body, usually a lower arm muscle, to test where the weakness in the body lies by touching various points on your body while exerting gentle pressure on your lower arm. He or she can determine exactly which HK procedures have to be carried out to help your system overcome this weakness so that you can get well again.

HK procedures can involve applying magnets to your body to correct a faulty electromagnetic field, your having to think a phrase or word, or test vials being placed on your body while various acupuncture points are being held.

Further information

BOOKS

Thurnell-Read, J. (2002) *Health Kinesiology*. Penzance: Life-Work Potential.

This book will give you very detailed information. The author is the longest-practising HK practitioner in the UK and brings a wealth of experience with her. Well written and highly recommended.

USEFUL ADDRESSES

Health Kinesiology UK
www.hk4health.co.uk
+44 (0)8707 655980

Kinesiology Federation
www.kinesiologyfederation.co.uk
+44 (0)845 260 1094

Treatment #3: Homeopathy

Homeopathy is based on the principle that a substance which produces certain symptoms in a healthy person will also cure a person who is ill and displays the same symptoms.

Homeopathy by now is a well established form of medicine. In the UK, there are a number of hospitals dedicated solely to homeopathy, with the National Health Service or private medical insurances paying for treatment if you are referred. There are also hundreds of fully qualified medical doctors who practise homeopathy today and even more lay homeopaths who have undergone rigorous training over several years to qualify.

Most homeopathic remedies are extracts of naturally occurring substances such as plants, animal material and natural chemicals. However, it is quite standard for homeopaths today also to use ordinary allopathic medicines in a highly diluted form to counteract any ill effects or damage the patient has sustained from using this medicine in the past.

The discovery of homeopathy goes back to Samuel Hahnemann, an 18th century German medical doctor. Hahnemann had become disillusioned with the medical approaches of his day when he stumbled across an interesting discovery. In Hahnemann's days, the bark of the cinchona tree was used to treat malaria. Hahnemann knew that one of the main symptoms of the disease was intermittent fevers, and he decided to experiment on himself. Without ever having suffered from malaria himself, he took multiple doses of cinchona for several days and noticed that he started coming out with intermittent fever. His explanation for this phenomenon was that the cinchona bark worked to cure malaria because it created an artificial illness in the body which resembled malaria and stimulated the body's defence mechanisms to combat the original disease.

Hahnemann, who had become a professor at Leipzig University, went on to study other plants and substances in a similar way, asking his students to take very small amounts of plant materials and keeping very detailed notes on how they affected them physically, emotionally and mentally. This process is called 'proving' a homeopathic remedy.

He collected all the information about the 'side-effects' of a plant when taken by a healthy individual and made up a homeopathic 'drug picture' from the data. He could now start matching his patients' symptoms to the side-effects of a plant. He then prescribed the plant and found that he was able to completely cure his patients of their diseases.

He found, however, that some patients were made worse by the normal dose of the plant, and so he started giving them the diluted form of the plant, thinking this would reduce the efficacy but would make it more tolerable to his patient. But rather than weakening the effect of the plant, he found to his surprise that the plant worked better but didn't have the unpleasant side-effects.

Since Hahnemann's times, many doctors and scientists have checked and rechecked Hahnemann's principles and found that they obtained the same excellent results with their patients.

What happens in a homeopathy session?

To start with, a homeopathic doctor will take a very detailed history from you, asking you about your illness and the medical aspects of it. In addition, you will have to answer questions about your personal life, your life-style, relationships, work and your likes and dislikes. This information is vital as the homeopath's choice of remedy will depend on your unique personal situation. Homeopathy is a highly individualised and holistic way of treating patients.

The homeopath will now choose a remedy that matches your illness most closely in its drug picture. In most cases, you will receive tiny tablets or pills which contain a highly diluted amount of the remedy. These are taken under the tongue until they have dissolved.

Homeopathic remedies should be taken on an empty stomach or at least ten minutes away from food. You will also be advised to avoid sweets, sugary foods, smoking and coffee.

Depending on the complexity of your health problem, you will be asked to return for another visit in four or more weeks. In your next consultation, your homeopath will want to find out how you have been and whether there have been any other symptoms that you have noticed. Your feedback will give the homeopath the necessary information to make up your new prescription. Imagine that with every visit, the homeopath is removing another layer of your illness until it is finally completely resolved.

Further information

BOOKS

Castro, M. (1990) *The Complete Homeopathy Handbook: A Guide to Everyday Health Care.* Kandern and Ioronto: Narayana Publishing.

A very useful book which describes the principles and concepts of homeopathy as well as listing a great number of homeopathic remedies. It also gives advice on self-prescription.

USEFUL ADDRESSES

The Society of Homeopaths
www.homeopathy-soh.org
+44 (0)845 450 6611

American Institute of Homeopathy
www.homeopathyusa.org
+1 888 445 9988

Australian Homeopathic Association
www.homeopathyoz.org
+61 07 4636 5081

NZ Homeopathic Society
http://homeopathy.ac.nz
+64 09 630 5458

Treatment #4: Dental orthopaedics

Depending on the problems you are having, it can be possible for a qualified dentist to spot the signs of a bite problem. Various muscles may be sore when tested, or the broken and worn areas of your teeth will show you are grinding your teeth – a common sign of an incorrect bite. There are now several options to correct this.

Tooth adjustment (equilibration)

Strictly speaking, this treatment is not an orthopaedic procedure as it does not change the shape of your jaw. I have included it here though because it helps heal the temporo-mandibular joint (TMJ). If your dentist suspects that your problems are due to an incorrect bite, they may help to diagnose the problem by supplying a temporary hard plastic splint that fits over your lower teeth. (The splint should not be fitted on the upper jaw as this can adversely affect movement of the cerebro-spinal fluid.)

This appliance needs to be measured and fitted very accurately so that when you bite on it, all your teeth meet at exactly the same time in a position where your muscles are relaxed. You may have to wear this all the time or just at night. If the appliance relieves your symptoms then your bite may need to be corrected permanently. This is achieved by minute adjustments to the enamel surfaces of your teeth.

Advanced Lightwire Functional (ALF)

This is the very latest in braces and is carried out by a dentist who has qualified in dental orthopaedics. Dental orthopaedics is different from orthodontics. Most of us know about orthodontics where you wear a fixed or removable brace to line up your teeth better. However, when you go for orthopaedic dentistry, you will have your upper jaw widened and/or teeth moved so that the TMJ is in the correct position. In order to achieve this, an ALF brace is used (there are also other types of braces which can be used).

The ALF appliance is made of a light, flexible wire which is looped around one of your back teeth and runs behind your teeth. This means it is invisible and does not affect your speech. ALF treats misaligned and malformed jaws as well as TMJ problems.

Dr Ljuba Lemke, a leading expert in ALF treatments who practises in Colorado and New Jersey in the United States, explains: 'A faulty bite can lead to misaligned vertebrae, leading to back, neck and shoulder problems. Also, nerves and blood vessels can become restricted so that there is decreased blood flow to the brain. A restricted movement of the jaw can lead to all sorts of problems such as digestive disorders, fatigue, PMS and many more'(private interview, 2005).

The bones in the head are not rigidly fused together. When you are healthy, there is a minute, rhythmic movement between the bones. When the bones of the skull are blocked up, the cerebro-spinal fluid cannot continue its movement to the brain, and this affects health as well as behaviour.

There are a number of causes for locked-up skull bones:

- trauma during birth, particularly when forceps are used

- injuries and accidents involving the head (whiplash)

- 'imitation' food which lacks nutrients and enzymes so that normal jaw development is repressed which in turn leads to crowding of teeth and an incorrect bite

- teeth loss without adequate replacement or severe tooth abrasion due to grinding or clenching

- dental treatment (extraction of wisdom teeth or teeth replacement) or orthodontic treatment which leaves the jaws in an unfavourable position.

If the bones of the head are locked up, cranial strain occurs which causes compromised function and more wear and tear. The effects are similar to those of a strained ankle: due to the pain the body tries to protect the injured part and comes up with compensatory mechanisms. As a consequence, other muscle groups are overused which leads to further problems.

The ALF brace corrects the cranial strain and enhances the rhythmic movement of the skull bones. In general, treatment times range between 18 to 48 months.

Replacement of teeth

The TMJ needs equal support from both sides of both jaws. The chewing action is designed to work properly only when all your teeth are present and in the correct position. Missing teeth may need to be replaced either with a partial denture or bridgework.

Replacement is not usually done until a diagnosis has been confirmed by using an appliance which fully relieves the symptoms. Relief in some patients is instant: in others it can take a long time – up to three months or more.

Diet and exercise

As with any joint pain, it can help to put less stress on the joint. A diet of soft foods can be helpful, as can corrective exercises and external heat. Physiotherapy exercises can often help (see earlier).

In order to find a dentist who can accurately assess your needs, look for a dentist who is qualified in dental orthopaedics or has qualifications in occlusal studies.

What happens in a dental orthopaedics session?

Your dentist may give you a questionnaire to check whether you have any allergies or intolerances, have had any accidents or operations and also whether you have any discomfort or pain anywhere in your body. This will give them an indication as to what is happening with the general alignment of your body.

If you go for ALF treatment, your dentist is also likely to send you for a number of x-rays to see the bone structure of your skull and find out where your jaw is compacted and which parts of the brain are compromised through the faulty bite. Then a number of casts of your teeth are taken, and sometimes also photographs of your face.

Avoid having an MRI scan though, unless it is absolutely necessary, as the gadolinium which is used for these scans can cause hair loss.

The exact type of treatment for your jaw will depend on the information gathered. Your dentist might recommend a fixed or a removable appliance.

Further information

BOOKS

Breiner, M.A. (1999) *Whole Body Dentistry: Discover the Missing Piece to Better Health.* Fairfield, CT: Quantum Health Press.

Explains about the dangers of various dental procedures, including orthodontics.

USEFUL INFORMATION

For information about TMJ alignment go to www.tmjstack.com.

For information about ALF treatment go to www.holistichealthsource.com.

For information about whole body dentistry go to www.WholeBodyDentistry.com.

To find a dentist who is qualified to adjust your bite contact:

The British Society for Occlusal Studies
www.bsos.co.uk

Dr Ljuba Lemke (Colorado)
www.HolisticHealthSource.com
+1 970 903 5128

Treatment #5: Hypnotherapy

Hypnotherapy has been practised in the UK for decades and has a very good track record for helping not only with psychological problems but also assisting in resolving physical matters. Studies have confirmed that learning self-hypnosis to relax can influence the body in a positive way so that self-healing can occur. Hypnotherapists have assisted their clients to get through tooth extractions or childbirth without painkillers and have also successfully taught those with unavoidable pain to anaesthetise their pain with the help of self-hypnosis.

Many illnesses are caused or made worse by psychological stresses or a stressful life-style, and hair loss is no exception. I have had two clients who only needed to learn how to relax properly, and their hair stopped falling out.

With hair loss, it is a chicken and egg situation. Are you losing your hair because you are stressed, or are you stressed because you are losing your hair? In either case, it makes a lot of sense to learn to relax deeply to give your body a chance to heal.

Sometimes matters can be more complicated though. Not everyone can overcome their stress by merely using positive images and visualisation (suggestion therapy). For some people, stress is a long established problem which dates back to past events in their lives, going all the way back to childhood. In this case, it is essential to sort out what happened in the past with the help of analytical hypnotherapy. Both suggestion therapy and analytical hypnotherapy involve hypnosis and should be carried out by a qualified hypnotherapist.

When you are in hypnosis, you are fully aware of what is going on. You will remember everything that is being said (provided you have a good memory) and you will simply feel very relaxed. At no point are you unconscious or under the control of the therapist. You can open your eyes any time you want to, but if your therapist is doing a good job, you'll feel very comfortable and will prefer to stay that way, with your eyes closed.

What happens in a hypnotherapy session?

At first, the hypnotherapist will spend some time with you talking about what you want to achieve and noting what exactly the problem is that you are coming to consult them for. Depending on whether you need suggestion therapy or analytical hypnotherapy, the process that now follows will be slightly different.

If you need suggestion therapy, the hypnotherapist will invite you to sit comfortably in an armchair which is often a recliner. Once you have closed your eyes, the therapist may take you through a relaxation exercise similar to the one described in Chapter 6, 'Remedy #5'. The tension and relaxing of muscles is called progressive muscle relaxation and is often a standard tool hypnotherapists use to help you relax physically and focus mentally.

Next, you might be given a pleasant, calming picture for your imagination. As you focus your attention on this image and visualise it as best you can, your mind starts relaxing and your body relaxes more. Once you are relaxed and comfortable, the hypnotherapist can start giving you the suggestions that are relevant to the aim you want to achieve.

If you need analytical hypnotherapy, your therapist may start in a similar way to help you relax physically and mentally, but then continue by asking you to speak about memories of events that were traumatic at the time. You can speak quite easily in hypnosis. Ideally, your therapist should help you work through those issues rather than just let you recall them. Releasing pent-up feelings and working through what has happened will have a great de-stressing effect on your body and your emotions.

Further information

BOOKS

Roet, B. (2000) *Understanding Hypnosis: A Practical Guide to the Health-giving Benefits of Hypnotherapy and Self-hypnosis.* London: Piatkus Books.

USEFUL ADDRESSES

UK

The Association for Professional Hypnosis and Psychotherapy
www.aphp.co.uk
+44 (0)1702 347691

USA

HMI Nationally Accredited College of Hypnotherapy
www.hypnosis.edu
+1 818 758 2730

CHAPTER 8

REGROWTH

What to Expect

Any practitioner who works ethically and is honest with you will not be able to guarantee that they can make your hair grow back. It is virtually a matter of keeping on going until you succeed.

It is also unrealistic to expect a quick fix. Hair can fall out very quickly, but it usually takes ages to grow back again. If hair loss is due to stress and you deal with altering your reactions to stress, then your hair loss will reverse relatively quickly, provided there are no other reasons for the hair loss. If you have lost all your hair as I had, it can take up to five years until the hair is more than a millimetre long and has colour.

When I look at all the men and women I have treated for hair loss over the last few years, I find that on the whole, men are easier to help than women. In most of the cases where I had a male client with a hair loss problem, I have been able to help within three to five sessions. Often, the hair loss stopped after only one to two sessions. One of my male clients came in the door for his initial consultation and showed me how many hairs came away if he just went through his hair with his fingers. At the end of his first health kinesiology session I asked him for a hair sample and he commented 'That will be easy!' going through his hair with his fingers, only to find that not a single hair had come out. We had to take a pair of scissors to cut off some hair.

On the whole, it takes considerably longer to help a woman with hair loss. In my opinion, this is because women have hormonal fluctuations, and these fluctuations are much more difficult to rebalance than those of men where hormones remain reasonably steady throughout their adult life. With women, it usually takes a good ten sessions, often more. Alopecia areata especially can be tricky. It is not that difficult to get the hair to regrow. The real challenge lies in stopping it from falling out again, and that means a great deal of detective work and constant rebalancing. With women, a great many more factors are involved than with men, and that makes treatment more time consuming and lengthy.

Checking progress

If you still have hair on your head you will notice improvements because the hair looks fuller and has more body.

If all the hair on your head has fallen out, you can check by looking at your scalp with a magnifying glass and a strong light behind you. When you check for hair, think *tiny*. The first vellus hairs can only be seen just above the surface of the skin in the margins of where the strong light shines onto the scalp.

Once you have started treatment, for example having your dental problems sorted out or going through a detox programme, give your scalp a year before expecting new hair growth.

What you will notice at a much earlier stage is that other health problems you have will start getting better, and about four months after getting your toxin levels down to nearly zero, you may also notice other positive improvements with your hair, so start looking out for the following:

- Hair colour looks darker. This means that nutrients are now getting to the hair.

- Less hair falls out than before, even though some hair still falls out.

- Hair feels fuller when you go through it with your hand or a comb.

- Hair has more body even though you can't see new growth.

- Hair looks bulkier even though you can't see new growth.

- Hair grows faster – you need to have it cut more often.

- Tiny new hairs are growing out of the previously empty follicles. These hairs may be colourless or have colour. Both are good and are signs of progress.

- New hair starts growing but breaks off. This means that nutrients are now beginning to get through to the hair, but not enough yet.

CHAPTER 9

WHAT TO DO UNTIL YOUR HAIR GROWS AGAIN

Until your hair grows back, you need to look after your scalp, even if no hair is growing on it at all. In addition, there are also ways in which you can help yourself look and feel better. There are quite a few products on the market today which can cover or disguise hair loss.

Masking hair loss

If your hair is very thin and the scalp shines through, there are quite a few brands of hair building fibres that you can apply to the scalp to make your hair look bulkier. The powders come in different colours – black, different browns, auburn, blond, grey and white – so that you can match them with your own hair colour. They are easy to apply and stay on all day.

There are different types of concealers, and you will have to try out which one suits you best.

Further information

Toppik
UK: www.hair123.co.uk
+44 (0)1424 797777
USA: www.toppik.com
+1 800 360 3046

DermMatch
UK: www.hairfantastic.co.uk
+44 (0)1302 863348

USA: www.dermmatch.com
+1 800 826 2824

Nanogen Nanofibres
UK: www.hairfantastic.co.uk
+44 (0)1302 863348
USA: www.nanothick.com
+1 626 821 0330

Wigs

I was extremely reluctant to buy a wig when my hair loss first started getting really serious. Buying a wig means admitting that you have a big problem with your hair, and we all prefer to think that it will all resolve itself in a few more weeks, so there is no need to get a hairpiece.

An important point to consider, though, is that you feel really terrible if half your hair is missing. Many people don't want to leave the house any more – they stop seeing friends and won't accept invitations because of how they look. If this is the case, it will only make matters worse. Not only do you have the upset about losing your hair, but you are also isolating yourself. It is really worth thinking about getting a wig, especially for women.

In all larger cities, you will find specialised shops that sell wigs. These shops will normally have a private cubicle where you can try on wigs without being disturbed by other customers. Some shops will charge you a nominal fee for trying on wigs, but this amount is reimbursed when you buy a wig. This is obviously to discourage people from trying on wigs for fun without any serious intention of buying one.

There are different types of wigs which can vary considerably in price.

Synthetic wigs

These are the ones you normally get in most wig shops. Depending on make and quality, they vary in price between £100 (USD $150) and £150 (USD $250), more if they are monofilament wigs in which case they can be up to £300 (USD $500).

The advantage of synthetic wigs is that they won't change shape in the rain and you can easily wash them yourself. You gently comb them through and then wash them with normal shampoo in cold water. Don't rub, don't pull, just leave the wig to soak for five minutes, then rinse with cold water. You then shake the wig out over the tub, pat it a bit drier with a towel, shake it again and then loosely sit it on the shampoo bottle to let it air-dry.

There are several types of synthetic wigs which have different caps. The cap is the base of the wig that sits on the head and is what the hair is attached to.

The standard cap is the most common and the most affordable type of wig cap. On a standard cap, the hair is machine-sewn onto the cap. The layers of hair on the cap are pre-designed into a particular style, and the crown of the cap is frequently crimped so that onlookers are unable to see through the hair and see the cap.

Another type of cap is the monofilament cap which incorporates a thin piece of material at the crown that is made of a see-through material into which the artificial hair is knotted. A monofilament wig looks very natural and is versatile. It can be styled in a variety of different ways because each hair on a monofilament cap is individually hand tied at the crown so that the hair can be brushed or parted in any direction. The monofilament cap is also soft and is more comfortable to wear than the conventional style wigs. Monofilament wigs are for people who have no hair and also come as toupees or partial hairpieces.

Another style is the lace front wig. These can be either made with synthetic hair, with human hair or with a mixture of both. A lace front wig has a see-through piece along the front hairline which is usually attached to your skin with glue. Alternatively, you can also have a piece of plastic behind the lace front and then use double-sided tape to attach it to your scalp. The advantage of a lace front wig is that, provided it is a good quality wig, your hairline looks very natural, so even if it gets windy and the wind blows the hair away from your forehead, you do not have to worry. The wig sits very securely on your head.

The disadvantage of synthetic wigs is that they will go frizzy if they get near heat sources. If, for example, you bend down to take things out of the oven while the oven is hot, it can ruin your wig after a few times. Also, any of the synthetic hair that touches the skin on your neck or your clothes is likely to start looking matted and frizzy after a while. You can, however, prolong the life of your wig if you comb out the back every night and spray some wig conditioner on it, then comb through it again with your fingers to separate the strands of hair.

Synthetic wigs will last between four and six months if you wear them every day. After that time, they start to look matted.

When you buy a wig, it is best to buy two at the same time so that you can change over to the new one whenever you need to. Make sure you buy your next wig straight away when you have started on your second one as your favourite style might be out of stock and need to be re-ordered. Wigs often come from the Far East, and getting a new one can take several weeks.

Human hair wigs

Many wig shops also have wigs made with human hair, although the selection is normally more limited than for synthetic ones. These wigs tend to be much more expensive.

The disadvantage of human hair wigs is that it is much more complicated to care for them as you need to treat them like real hair and restyle them after washing. The colour can also fade if you spend a lot of time in the sun so that you may have to dye them again. They also need to be fitted well to your head, so remember to sew a piece of thin plastic into the front (unless the wig has that already) and use double-sided tape to secure it to your scalp.

TIPS

- Don't buy wigs with a fixed parting. They never look natural.

- Some hairdressers will cut a wig for you to get as close as possible to your usual style. Find out by ringing a few salons to see whether one of the stylists can do this for you. If you are near London, contact Trevor Sorbie's salon (www.trevorsorbie. com) where there are stylists who specialise in cutting wigs.

- Go to a wig shop for your first wig and let someone explain how to wear it correctly, how to alter the size, etc. Once you have your first wig, start looking on the internet for the same wig. You can often get the same wig cheaper over the internet.

- To hold a synthetic wig in place, sew a little patch of plastic into the front of the wig and use special double sided adhesive strips (from wig suppliers) to fasten the wig to your scalp. That way you will feel more secure when there is a wind.

- If you want to use a hairspray on your wig, make sure it is one that does not do damage to your scalp. I recommend Jason's Thin-to-Thick hairspray.

Vacuum wigs

If you can afford it, these are the very best wigs. They are shaped exactly to your head and have the same advantages as the monofilament with an added advantage. They actually stick to your head by suction which makes them totally secure to wear. The price reflects all the work that goes into them – you will have to spend at least £1500 (USD $2500) on this type of wig.

Vacuum wigs are made with human hair. To get a vacuum wig, you will need to go for several visits. Initially, you will have to spend two to three hours so that a plaster mould of your scalp can be made. You will then have to return for another visit to check that the wig base fits perfectly and to choose the hair colour you want. At the third visit, you will be able to try on the wig and have it styled to your exact specifications.

The advantage of a vacuum wig is that you can do virtually anything in it. It is very easy to put on and take off, and no matter how windy it is outside, you can always be sure your wig stays firmly on your head. You can go to the hairdressers and have the wig washed and styled on your head, and you can go swimming in it without any problems. This wig will last you for about two to three years.

Vacuum wigs will only fit securely if you have no hair at all or if you are prepared to shave off any remaining hair and keep it shaved off. The suction will not work properly if you have hair.

Sue is the UK supplier of vacuum wigs which originally come from New Zealand and are also available in the USA and Australia. Sue works from the privacy of her own home in a relaxed and private atmosphere. She has many years of experience with wigs and can also advise you on other types of wigs and hairpieces.

Further information

WIGS AND HATS

Vacuum wigs from Sue Renigan
www.positivelyhair.co.uk
+44 (0)1993 811 880

If you don't want to go for a wig, you can also go for a turban if you are a woman.
www.freedomwigs.com/contact-us
(You will find telephone numbers for each country in this section.)

www.2ndnaturehair.com/about

www.realityhair.ca
+1 403 226 8585

Luscious Lids
www.lusciouslids.com
+44 (0)23 8084 8687

Hats and Hair
www.hatsandhair.co.uk
+44 (0)871 662 9302

Hats and scarves
www.hatsscarvesandmore.com
+1 877 838 6151

Jason's Thin to Thick hairspray
www.JasonNaturalCare.co.uk

Extensions

Another option for women with thinning hair is getting extensions. These are woven or heat-bound into your own hair which means that your hair will have to have a minimum length to support the extension. These days, the extension techniques are quite advanced so that even fairly short hair can have extensions attached.

The advantages of extensions are that you feel more natural than if you wear a wig. There is nothing 'on' your head, but your hair is simply longer and looks fuller which will make you feel more confident.

The disadvantages are that the extensions need to be fastened to your own hair quite tightly if they are woven in and might make more hair fall out through the traction (see also traction alopecia in Chapter 1). Also, you will need to have the extensions re-done approximately every six weeks which makes it a bit expensive for some people. For the money you spend on one extension treatment, you can get a wig that will last you four to six months if you look after it well. However, many women are happier with extensions because they find it difficult to take the big step of wearing a wig.

An alternative to woven-in extensions are protein bonded extensions. These are fastened to a strand of your hair with a tool that bonds the artificial strand to your hair through heat. These extensions are much faster to put in than the woven extensions and can stay in the hair for up to three months. They also don't put the strain on your own hair as the woven extensions do.

Eyebrows and eye definition

If you have had the misfortune of losing not only the hair on your head but also your eyebrows and eyelashes, you may feel as though you are left with no face. It is amazing how much definition eyebrows and eyelashes give the face, even if you don't accentuate them with mascara and an eyebrow pencil.

Eyebrows

The simplest way to replace your eyebrows is to draw on eyebrows using an eyebrow pencil and some liquid eyeliner (*not* a permanent one). Make sure the colour is not too dark. If your hair or wig colour is brown, don't buy a black eyebrow pencil and eyeliner, as this will look too stark.

First, put a little powder over your eyebrow area unless your skin is quite dry anyway. If your skin is greasy, the eyebrows you draw will get smudged, especially if your hairpiece comes down to the eyebrow line. Next, draw a light line with the eyebrow pencil where you want your eyebrows to be. Feather the line a little with small pencil strokes that go upwards. Now put some liquid eyeliner onto a surface, maybe the edge of your mirror. Dilute it slightly with some water. Now go over the pencilled eyebrow shapes again with little strokes and let the eyeliner dry.

By using an eyeliner over the pencil, your eyebrows will last much longer through the day. Eyebrow pencil on its own will quickly grease up and get smeared.

Another option is to use transfer eyebrows which act like a temporary tattoo. These are very nice, look very real and don't rub off easily, as long as you keep your moisturising and cleanser creams away from them when you put make-up on or take it off. These eyebrows last between three and seven days, depending on how oily your skin is.

To put them onto your eyebrow area, cut out the eyebrow and detach the see-through plastic film. Put the eyebrow into the right place, then gently press a wet cloth onto the eyebrow transfer for about a minute. You can then take off the cloth and peel off the remaining plastic and, hey presto, you have a beautifully shaped eyebrow which you don't have to pluck!

Tips

- Always make sure that your skin is clean and your eyebrow area has no moisturiser on it before you place the eyebrows.

- Put both eyebrows on together to make sure they are at the same height and the same distance away from the midline of your face.

- Don't bother buying a very expensive band to hold the eyebrows in place while you are transferring them onto your skin. It's a waste of money. Fold up a couple of pieces of toilet paper and run water over them; that works just as well!

- If you use very warm water, the eyebrows transfer much more quickly.

- You can go swimming with the eyebrows; just make sure you don't rub your towel over them afterwards. Just let your forehead dry by itself and they will last you longer.

Further information

Beauti-Full-Brows:
UK: www.wigsandpieces.com
+44 (0)1964 631199
USA: www.beauti-full-brows.com
+1 800 241 1598

Both websites have a very helpful video which shows you how to put on the eyebrows.

If you want something more permanent, you can go for semi-permanent make-up, also known as tattoo make-up. This is imprinted into the skin where your eyebrows should be. This will last for several years. It's also good if you simply want to define your eyebrows more because you don't have much eyebrow hair growing.

Some of my clients found the process a bit painful, though, so if you are squeamish, you'll probably be much happier with the transfer eyebrows.

If you go for this option, choose mineral colours over plant colours. Mineral colours tend to stay more stable whereas plant colours can change a bit more from the original colour over time.

To find someone near you, Google 'semi-permanent make-up'.

Eye definition

For definition of the eyes, you can simply get a soft kajal pencil and outline the upper eyelid and the lower one. Once you have done that, go over those lines with a gel eyeliner to make it last better throughout the day. Do check every once in a while though to make sure you still have a defined outline, and always carry some gel eyeliner with you. If you are fair-skinned, use brown rather than black kajal and eyeliner, otherwise the lines look too harsh.

Or you may want to consider semi-permanent make-up as described in the eyebrow section earlier on.

Another option is to get fine strip lashes. Make sure they don't have any fancy pattern where they attach to the strip. The more natural they look, the more comfortable you will feel in them.

If necessary, cut the lashes shorter with nail scissors by trimming the entire length of the hairs shorter. Then go over them again and shorten every third hair a little more to make them look less even.

Hold each strip lash to the appropriate eye and cut the length of the strip according to how big your upper or lower eye line is.

Rather than using the adhesive that comes with the eyelashes (which is normally not very good), buy Duo Adhesive which you can get at the Mac cosmetic counter in your local department store or, if you can get it in the UK, the Ardell LashGrip Adhesive which is the best in my experience. Apply a thin line of adhesive onto the strip lashes and wait for 15 seconds to let it go tacky. Next, holding the strip with both hands, gently put it onto your eyeline where your lashes would normally be.

Keep the strip lashes in place for a moment and then move them until they are in exactly the right place. Make sure the lashes don't droop down over your eye but hold them in place with your finger so that they are turned upwards a bit to give a natural look.

Whenever you can, don't use false eyelashes as the adhesive is not particularly good for your skin, so if you can go without them on a day off or on a weekend, take the opportunity to give your body a break from the glue.

If you want a natural look, go for No. 107 or No. 070 Eylure upper lashes and No. 020 for lower lashes. These are available at Boots Pharmacy in the UK, at many drugstores in the USA or over the internet.

CHAPTER 10

THE FEEL-GOOD SECTION

People who Got Their Hair Back Using Natural Methods

Here are some of the case histories of people who have regained their hair through health kinesiology (HK), taking supplements after hair/nail sample testing or through other natural means.

One of my clients told me about her aunt who noticed how her hair was beginning to thin when she was in her sixties. The aunt began immediately to brush her hair vigorously several times a day and managed to get her full head of hair back well into her eighties.

*

'I now have hair growth which is coming in as you said at our last appointment.' [Female client, 23]

*

A male client, aged 62, came to me for hair loss problems. He had noticed how his hair had started falling out a lot during washing which was unusual for him as he had a very good full head of hair. After three sessions of health kinesiology, his hair loss had stopped and after a further three weeks he noticed that his hair looked fuller.

*

'Hair starting to grow back slowly, can see improvement. Digestion has improved after new diet, much less diarrhoea. Scalp is better.' [This was after nine weeks on the supplements and food exclusions that were tested with the big hair sample test.]

*

A young woman in her early thirties came to see me with total hair loss on the entire body (alopecia universalis). This had occurred after part of her thyroid had been destroyed in a medical procedure which was supposed to cure her overactive thyroid. As a consequence, she now had an underactive thyroid and had lost all her hair overnight. We started health kinesiology treatment and found that her body was unable to recognise and metabolise a number of important nutrients. We corrected this through a number of health kinesiology procedures, and after ten sessions, her hair started growing again.

*

[From 31-year-old male client, sent in 11 weeks after having done the first hair sample test and taking the supplements prescribed] 'Dramatic improvement with only a few hairs in the shower every morning. My previous [hair] sample was easily obtained by simply brushing my hair prior to showering; this one [hair sample] had to be cut!'

*

An acquaintance, a middle-aged lady in her late forties, told me how she had started losing her hair in round patches (alopecia areata) about ten years ago. As her doctor did not seem to have any solutions, she decided to consult a homeopath to see if she could help.

The homeopath found out that the hair loss problem was due to a number of vaccinations the client had had for her travels to the Far East, as well as a prolonged period of great stress in her personal life. She prescribed homeopathic remedies, and the client had to return for a number of visits approximately six to eight weeks apart, but finally, the hair grew back without a recurrence of the problem.

*

'Have just washed my hair and no hair was falling out. Went to see the beautician yesterday to have my eyelashes tinted and eyebrows shaped. She commented that my eyelashes were a lot thicker now when before they had always been very thin. I also noticed that I have thicker hairs on my scalp.' [German female client, 40]

*

A young woman of 27 came with very serious hair loss which she had had for eight years ever since she had a very stressful period as an au pair abroad. Her hair had always been fine, but now the scalp was shining through everywhere. Her hairs were like wisps. We had to work with health kinesiology for about 13 sessions until her hair started looking darker and thicker. When she came in for her last session, the difference was quite visible, and her hairdresser had also remarked on how her hair had improved.

*

A male Asian client came very distressed because his formerly full hair had been reduced to half the volume he had before. His hair was coming out when he was washing it, and he would always find hair on his pillow in the morning. He couldn't understand why this was happening – nobody in his family had problems with their hair. In addition, he also suffered from irritable bowel syndrome. On checking with my foods test kit, I found that he had multiple allergies and had to stay away from some foods which he ate a lot of. He had already stopped smoking and now also stopped drinking as he proved to be intolerant to every kind of alcohol. Once he had made these adjustments, the hair stopped falling out. With a couple more health kinesiology sessions, his hair quality started improving and the hair started looking denser again.

*

[From an US female client who has had 12 years of severe telogen effluvium] 'I see lots of little hairs poking out all over my head. Definitely thicker and in great shape. The sides have really thickened up.'

*

A client of 60 came with a number of health problems. She suffered from diabetes, rheumatoid arthritis, irritable bowel, panic attacks, anxiety and alopecia areata. With health kinesiology treatment, the hair started growing but kept falling out again and again. She had a great number of crowns in her mouth which had been put in a long time ago. At first my client was very reluctant to go to a dentist as this would have meant financial outlay for having the crowns with the amalgam inside removed and replaced. However, when her own dentist told her that some of the crowns needed replacing anyway, I was able to persuade her to see the dentist I work with who specialises in amalgam removal. He found that there was an area of serious inflammation in her jaw, and on removing one of the crowns found that it had amalgam inside. Gradually, she had all the crowns with amalgam replaced and the difference in her hair growth became quickly apparent. The hair started growing better and more quickly, without it falling out again.

*

'I will be posting another hair sample to you tomorrow and I am pleased to say that my hair is looking better and does not seem to be shedding as much.' [Male client, 27]

*

A young man of 24 came to see me. He had had problems with his hair since the age of 14 when he had developed thinning hair on his crown. He was eating a lot of junk food, drank lots of diet coke and was also very dehydrated. We started with a little tidy-up of his diet by reducing the junk food somewhat and increasing water intake.

At the same time, eight sessions of health kinesiology were necessary to allow his body to rebalance itself and allow nutrients to get into the cells. At his last session, he came back, sporting a shorter hairstyle and showing off a clearly denser hair growth than he had had before.

*

'I have taken the drops and supplements you tested for me. My skin has improved and I have noticed my mind feels a lot clearer, my memory has improved and I feel much less stressed. The scabs on my head are slowly going. I had two verrucas on my right foot which I have had for about six years. About two weeks after starting the supplements they just fell off.' [Male client, 33]

*

'After the hair sample test, I started taking the supplements that you had tested for me. After only eight weeks, my hair had improved dramatically. It is shinier, in better condition and more manageable and it feels less thin on my scalp which has lost its former angry redness. The scalp feels more relaxed, the hair also feels stronger and has more life in it, is less porous and less frizzy – taking much longer to dry after shampooing because there is more of it.' [Female client from Germany, 42]

*

When I spoke in a radio programme about the success I've had with my health kinesiology treatment for men and women with hair loss problems, a man rang in to say that he had started losing his hair a year ago but that a friend had suggested he used apple cider vinegar. He had applied it twice every day and his hair grew back again.

*

'Just thought you might like to have some feedback. At the beginning of September this year you did a hair analysis for me and recommended some supplements which I have now been taking for about ten weeks.

I went to the hairdresser today. I still have hair integration around my crown but I had noticed that my own hair at the back and sides seemed to have improved in texture. I thought perhaps I was imagining it because it is what I want to believe. The girl who did my hair today last did it three months ago. She asked if I had noticed a difference in my hair. I said that I had and what did she think the difference was. She said the texture is much better and it appears to be getting thicker. I am delighted because she must have noticed a significant difference to comment. I feel for the first time in almost ten years (which is when my hair first started falling) that just maybe I will beat this and in time be able to dispense with the integration. The other thing that I have noticed is that when I run my hands through my hair it doesn't come out.'

*

'I was going to write to you on Saturday already, but I guess I was too busy celebrating :-) I had this feeling that something was different for the last week or so, and my mum when she saw me last week mentioned how much longer and thicker my hair was… I haven't been examining my hair and scalp much lately because when I would do so in the past, I would only see the hair that I did not have, and that was so frustrating all the time…but on Saturday afternoon I felt I should really check what is going on – and after a ten-minute investigation in front of a mirror I had to conclude without a doubt that my hair got thicker! (On Friday, the day before, it was exactly six months since I started taking your supplements for the first time.) When I part it there's not so much skin visible, it looks just normal, and just now I took the time to part it in the middle of my head again and then fix it with two pins on the side and hold together the rest of the hair at the back of my head – and it looked good, no scalp showing through! And I also parted it from my forehead all the way back to my neck and tied it behind both ears, and that looks good too.' [Female client in Hungary, 32]

*

After six weeks on the supplements prescribed as a result of the hair sample test, this 29-year-old male client reports: 'Less hair loss. Some new hair. Skin around hair follicles seems a bit stronger. Generally feeling much better and positive overall. Scalp less itchy.'

*

'This is to thank you for Wednesday's session. I slept well that night and in fact have had a run of good sleeps since with no spontaneous waking. Something is working here. Hair loss has pretty much stopped for a few weeks now. Oh, and a cut in my ear that kept seeping and hadn't healed properly for 18 months looks like it might be healing properly now.'

*

'I just thought you would like to know the progress with my hair. Over the past five weeks I have seen tremendous results; my hair has stopped falling to as little as 10 to 30 hairs when I wash and dry it. Before, my hair used to cover the floor of my bedroom, now I can only see a few. My scalp is less greasy, it used to be very greasy, even on the day I washed it, within hours it would become greasy, now I only need to wash every two or three days apart. I have after your analysis cut out sugar, cow's milk and wheat radically.'

*

'Overall, I can report that something must have shifted when I did the detox as per your hair sample test. My eyebrows are growing again as well as the eyelashes. The skin on my face is beautifully clear and no longer so very dry. My scalp has become more "open" and does not seem to be so shiny any more and my hair has more body. Overall, my hair has become stronger. When I run my fingers over my scalp, I can feel hair and not bald, tense scalp as I used to. My scalp has also become more flexible and I can shift it to and fro more easily! In the middle bit on top of my head there are now a few new hairs. The hair loss has stopped. The itchiness has gone completely.' [From a German female client]

*

'Not only has my hair started growing again, but my scalp is now totally normal and no longer flaky and dry, and the acne on my back has also disappeared. Doing the hair sample test and taking the supplements has been worth every penny, and I would recommend it to anyone with a hair loss problem!' [Male client]

*

'I went to my hairdressers the other day and made a point of not saying anything about my hair, so his remark was unprompted. He said to me, "I don't know what you are doing, but your hair is in very good condition and it is regrowing!" I'm really pleased with how much better my hair is growing after only three months of health kinesiology treatment.'

*

The treatment even works for animals! Diane contacted me to say that her cat Barney had lost nearly all the hair along his spine because he was overgrooming (constant licking over the area). This had been going on for two years, and the vet did not know what to do about it. Diane sent me a hair sample of Barney and as I tested it, I found that the overgrooming was a stress reaction. Barney must have had a shock, maybe a near accident, which made him become obsessive about grooming. I was able to test which homeopathic remedy was necessary to help him overcome the shock. Diane put one drop of the remedy on Barney's food every night, and after four weeks, all the fur had regrown and Barney had stopped overgrooming. Psychotherapy with homeopathic drops!

*

A 47-year-old lady came to see me for health kinesiology. She had been having problems with her hair since giving birth to her third child, and over the last five years she had lost a lot of hair. Conventional therapy with minoxidil made even more hair fall out, and iron supplementation prescribed by a hair specialist only resulted in limited improvement of her diffuse hair loss. When I checked her, it turned out that she had two amalgam and one gold filling. I explained to her that this is a particularly bad combination as the different metals create currents in the mouth that disturb the body's functioning. My client had the amalgam fillings changed for white fillings and we tested for the right detoxifying herbs for her to take for six weeks after the dental treatment. After a couple of health kinesiology sessions, her hair was visibly darker and fuller. She does not have to take any iron supplements any more as the health kinesiology helped her body to correctly metabolise iron from the food she is eating.

*

And here is a recent e-mail from one of my clients who had been on a treatment plan which I had put together for her after having carried out a hair sample test: 'Hello Vera, :-))))) I am so so so pleased!!! Thank you very much for my results and all your help I feel amazing and am so grateful. I wasn't expecting my mercury levels to be clear or the fungus to be dead. I'm ecstatic at the news. Finally seeing hair growth that seems to be staying put just shows me my system needed an overhaul and I am so pleased the universe sent you as my gift!'

Final words

Well, now you know a lot of what I know. As you can see there is truly no quick fix to getting your hair back, but there are ways of helping it regrow. Many of my clients who did not want chemicals in their body or on their scalp have had success with one or several of the methods that I have presented in this book.

I personally think that it is important to work with the body and not against it. You can't force hair to grow back; you can only help the body get rid of toxins and stock up on the essential nutrients. Once the body is back in balance, hair can regrow. While you are working at getting your hair to regrow naturally, you will also sort out a few other health problems you may not even have been aware of.

Always remember that by the time your hair starts falling out, a lot has already gone wrong in your body. Even though it is possible to lose hair as a consequence of one serious shock, in most cases, hair loss is the result of a long-term problem that won't allow the body to stay in balance any more. For you, this means that you need to find the reason why your hair can't grow any more. To do that, you may need to consult a practitioner. It may take a while until you have discovered why it happened in the first place, but once you know, there are natural treatments and remedies that can redress the balance.

If you feel you are losing all hope, please read through the case histories in the previous chapter again.

Please don't give up. It is never too late. Take me as an example. If my hair can start growing again after 30 years, there is no reason why yours shouldn't.

Other than that, do get on with your life. Don't let your lack of hair stop you from living. I have always had boyfriends who didn't care about my lack of hair. I got on with my job and eventually set up a successful practice. I have always had good friends who couldn't have cared less whether I had hair or not. If I can do it, you can do it too. Get cracking, get going, deal with the problem and live your life to the full. There's lots to do – let's not be held back by a lack of hair!

Contact details
For appointments

+44 (0)1252 501050
Email hairgrowth@peiffer.co.uk
Telephone consultations by arrangement.
Skype consultations by arrangement.
For more information on fees, please see
www.hairgrowthUK.net ('Services' section.)

BIBLIOGRAPHY

Andrew, A.S., Schned, A.R., Heaney, J.A. and Karaga, M.R. (2004) 'Bladder cancer risk and personal hair dye use.' *International Journal of Cancer 109*, 4, 581–588.

Banerjee, A., Pathak, S., Biswas, S., Roy-Karmakar, S., et al. (2010) '30C and 200C in induced hepato-toxicity in rats. *Homeopathy,* 99, 3, 167-76.

Bartram, T. (1998) *Bartram's Encyclopedia of Herbal Medicine.* London: Robinsons.

Björkman, L., Lundekvam, B.F., Laegreld, T., Bertelsen BI et al. (2007) 'Mercury in human brain, blood, muscle and toenails in relation to exposure: an autopsy study.' *Environmental Health 6*, 30.

Braverman, E.R. with Pfeiffer, C.C., Blum, K. and Smayda, R. (1997) *The Healing Nutrients Within.* Canaan, CT: Keats Publishing.

British Dental Association (2007) Dental Waste Disposal. Available from www. dentalwastedisposal.co.uk/pdf/BritishDenta07.pdf, accessed on 11 December 2012.

Budd, M. (2000) *Why Am I So Tired? Is Your Thyroid Making You Ill?* London: Thorsons.

Dhillon S., von Burg R. (1995) 'Isopropyl Alcohol.' *Journal of Applied Toxicology 15*, 6, 501–506.

Ericson, A. and Källen, B. (1989) 'Pregnancy outcome in women working as dentists, dental assistants or dental technicians.' *International Archives of Occupational and Environmental Health 61*, 5, 329–333.

Fulgenzi, A., Zanella, S.G., Mariani, M.M., Vietti, D. and Ferrero, M.E. (2012) 'A case of multiple sclerosis improvement following removal of heavy metal intoxication: lessons learnt from Matteo's case.' *Biometals 25*, 3, 569–576.

Gründling C., Schimetta W., Frass, M. (2012) 'Real-life effect of classical homeopathy in the treatment of allergies: *A multicenter prospective observational study.' Wien Klin ochenschr 124*, 1-2, 11-7.

Health and Safety Executive (2002) Control of Substances Hazardous to Health. Available from www.hse.gov.uk/nanotechnology/coshh.htm, accessed on 11 December 2012.

Huggins, H.A. (1993) *It's All in Your Head. The Link between Mercury Amalgams and Illness.* New York: Avery Publishing.

Johannson, B.I. (1986a) 'Electrochemical action due to short-circuiting of dental alloys. An in vitro and in vivo study.' *Swedish Dental Journal Supplement 33*, 1–47.

Johannson, B.I. (1986b) 'Tin and copper release related to charge transfer between short-circuited amalgam and gold alloy electrodes.' *Scandinavian Journal of Dental Research 94*, 3, 250–266.

Lindh, U., Danersund, A. and Lindvall, A. (1996) 'Selenium protection against toxicity from cadmium and mercury studied at the cellular level.' *Cellular and Molecular Biology (Noisy-le-grand) 42*, 1, 39–48.

Khuda-Bukhsh, A., Banerjee, A., Biswas, S., Karmakar, S., Banerjee, P., et al. (2011) 'An initial report on the efficacy of a millesimal potency rsenicum Album LM 0/3 in ameliorating arsenic toxicity in humans living in a high-risk arsenic village.' *Zhong Xi Yi Jie He Xue Bao 9*, 6, 596-604.

McTaggart, L. (2003) *Your Healthy House.* London: WDDTY Publication.

McTaggart, L. (2005) *What Doctors Don't Tell You.* London: HarperCollins.

McTaggart, L. (2006) *The WDDTY Dental Handbook.* London: WDDTY Publication.

Mamede, A.C., Pires, A.S., Abrantes, A.M., Tavares, S.D. et al. (2012) 'Cytotoxicity of ascorbic acid in a human colorectal adenocarcinoma cell line (WiDr): in vitro and in vivo studies.' *Nutritional Cancer 64*, 7, 1049–1057.

Matte, T.D., Mulinare, J. and Erickson, J.D. (1993) 'Case control study of congenital defects and parental employment in health care.' *American Journal of Industrial Medicine 24*, 1, 11–23.

McComb, D. (1997) 'Occupational exposure to mercury in dentistry and dentist mortality.' *Journal of the Canadian Dental Association 63*, 5, 372–376.

Mervyn, L. (1989) *Thorsons Complete Guide to Vitamins and Minerals.* London: Thorsons.

Naude, D., Couchman, S., Maharaj, A. (2010) 'Chronic primary insomnia: Efficacy of homeopathic simillimum.' *Homeopathy*, 99, 1, 63-8.

Peraza, M.A., Ayala-Fierro, F., Barber, D.S., Casarez, E. and Rael, L.T. (1998) 'Effects of micronutrients on metal toxicity.' *Environmental Health Perspectives 106*, Suppl 1, 203–216.

Pfeiffer, V. (2003) Total Stress Relief. *Practical Solutions that Really Work.* London: Piatkus.

Psarras, V., Derand, T. and Nilner, K. (1994) 'Effect of selenium on mercury vapour released from dental amalgams: an in vitro study.' *Swedish Dental Journal 18*, 1–2, 15–23.

Rowland, A.S., Baird, D.D., Weinberg, C.R., Shore, D.L., Shy, C.M. and Wilcox, A.J. (1994) 'The effect of occupational exposure to mercury vapour on the fertility of female dental assistants.' *Occupational and Environmental Medicine 51*, 1, 28–34.

Sancho, F.M. and Ruiz, C.N. (2010) 'Risk of suicide amongst dentists: myth or reality?' *International Dental Journal 60*, 6, 411–418.

Shafer, N. and Shafer, R.W. (1976) 'Potential carcinogenic effects of hair dyes.' *New York State Journal of Medicine 76*, 394–396.

Shore, R.E., Pasternack, B.S. Thiessen, E.U., Sadow, M., Forbes, R. and Albert, R.E. (1979) 'A case-control study of hair dye use and breast cancer.' *Journal of the National Cancer Institute 62*, 277–283.

Sikorski, R., Juszkiewicz, T., Paszkowski, T. and Szprengier-Juszkiewicz, T. (1987) 'Women in dental surgeries: reproductive hazards in occupational exposure to metallic mercury.' *International Archives of Occupational and Environmental Health 59*, 6, 551–557.

Siblerud, R.L. and Kienholz, E. (1994) 'Evidence that mercury from silver dental fillings may be an etiological factor in multiple sclerosis.' *Science of the Total Environment 142*, 3, 191–205.

Stanbury, R.M. and Graham, E.M. (2008) 'Systemic corticosteroid therapy – side effects and their management.' *British Journal of Ophthalmology 82*, 704¬–708.

Summers, A.O., Wireman, J., Vimy, M.J., Lorscheider, F.L. et al. (1993) 'Mercury released from dental 'silver' fillings provokes an increase in mercury- and antibiotic-resistant bacteria in oral and intestinal floras of primates.' *Antimicrobial Agents in Chemotherapy 37*, 4, 825–834.

World Health Organization (1990) 'International Programme on Chemical Safety: environmental health criteria.' *Inorganic Chemistry 118*, 61.

World Health Organization (2003) Concise International Chemical Assessment Document 50. Elemental Mercury and Inorganic Mercury Compounds: Human Health Aspects. Available from http://www.who.int/ipcs/publications/cicad/en/cicad50.pdf, accessed on 11 December 2012.

World Health Organization (2008) Guidelines for Identifying Populations at Risk from Mercury Exposure. Available from www.who.int/foodsafety/publications/chem/mercury/en/, accessed on 11 December 2012.

Wu, Y.H., Chuang, S.Y., Hong, W.C., Lai, Y.J., Chang, G.J. and Pang, J.H. (2012) 'Berberine reduces leukocyte adhesion to LPS stimulated endothelial cells and VCAM-1 expression both in vivo and in vitro.' *International Journal of Immunopathology and Pharmacology 25*, 3, 741–750.

Yan, L., Yan, K., Kun, W., Xu, L. et al. (2012) 'Berberine inhibits the migration and invasion of T24 bladder cancer cells via reducing the expression of heparanase.' Tumour Biology, epub ahead of print.

Ziemba, S.E., Menard, S.L., McCabe, M.L. Jr and Rosenspire, A.J. (2009) 'T-cell receptor signaling is mediated by transient Lck activity, which is inhibited by inorganic mercury.' *The FASEB Journal 23*, 1663–1671.

INDEX